Wendy Nordick holds a PhD and practiced social work for 25 years in acute care psychiatry and mental health in Kamloops, British Columbia, Canada. She has published academic journal articles and is a member of a local writing group. She is a lover of literature. As a life-long learner, she is tackling the intricacies of bridge, and meets her need for fresh air with skiing, pickleball, cycling and hiking. She and her husband, Bill, love adventure and have visited more than 40 countries. Scuba diving is a thrilling aspect of their travels. A mother of five children and two stepchildren, she delights in her 11 grandchildren.

Wendy Nordick

INDELIBLE: A SOCIAL WORKER IN THE WAKE OF CIVIL WAR

AUSTIN MACAULEY PUBLISHERS™

LONDON • CAMBRIDGE • NEW YORK • SHARJAH

A CIP catalogue record for this title is available from the British Library.

ISBN 9781398439146 (Paperback)
ISBN 9781398441309 (ePub e-book)

www.austinmacauley.com

First Published 2023
Austin Macauley Publishers Ltd®
1 Canada Square
Canary Wharf
London
E14 5AA

Table of Contents

Prologue

Feelings of inadequacy are often the steep stairs to heaven.

I stumbled on the chapel by accident. I found it one morning while I was out for my daily run. I used my runs to explore the areas of Jaffna, Sri Lanka and each day I chartered a different course. One day, shortly after arriving in Jaffna, I headed northeast from my house to explore a small area known as Chundikuli.

I spied a tiny church that appeared sunk in the red mud and I ventured towards it, careful not to twist an ankle in the deep, semi-dried ruts. Curious, I mounted the two steps to the entrance and crossed the threshold of the chapel, moving out of the blistering sunlight into the coolness of the shade inside. I looked around.

Bird droppings splattered the flooring at the wide entrance of the chapel where no door hung. Gaudy plastic flowers stood in vases, oblivious to the layers of dust twisting them into a tired gesture. The chapel was devoid of pews. I assumed the worshipers must sit on the concrete floor while listening to the Holy Mass. Despite being a Catholic, I was a stranger here and felt like an interloper.

I knelt upon the red, roughly cemented floor in front of the uncloaked wooden altar. A gentle, musky sea breeze fluttered off the shallow lagoon and in through the open soffits along the ceiling. I felt the fine, damp blond hairs on my arms lift by an unseen puff of air.

Strung from a brass hook twisted into the ceiling of the chapel, a sisal macramé hanger held a lonely candle with a flame sputtering to stay alive in the breeze. The candle wax had morphed into a misshapen lump, spilling onto splintered pottery dish sunk into the well of the hanger. I knew that a burning candle indicated the presence of the Blessed Sacrament, although the chapel seemed devoid of a tabernacle, the place where the host is stored.

A statue of the Virgin Mary, painted in stark primary, colours was sandwiched between the plastic flowers. Her iris-less eyes were devoid of emotion, recognition, or encouragement. She was not the Virgin Mary I held in my mind's eye.

9

I gazed out the window space. Mounted in the characteristic red mud of the island, a statue of Blessed Joseph Vaz stood like a sentinel between the sea and the chapel. I had read that Vaz was a Catholic priest from Goa who brought Christianity to many Sinhalese and Tamil people. He was the patron saint of Sri Lanka and statues of him dot churchyards across the island.

I mused as I knelt. Like me, he must have struggled with the Sinhala and Tamil languages. I imagined how different the cultures must have seemed to him, in a time long before global travel. I felt a kinship with the priest. He brought Christianity to the country while I was trying to bring better mental health to the country. Did he feel the same helplessness that I felt? Then, even from my kneeling position, I watched as a black cormorant winged by, landing on the priest's head. The bird teetered, then shat on the holy man's statue. "Naughty bird," I laughed, shifting my gaze back inside.

Behind the simple altar stood a giant wooden cross, dwarfing the whole chapel. Upon this cross hung a plaster version of the crucified Christ. Orangey red paint dribbled from the wound in His side and rusty red paint spattered His hands and feet. His head, stapled with long black thorns, dripped black blood into brown eyes drooping in pain.

Stark. Bloody. In North America, many churches prefer to portray the risen Christ, all white and pure and transfigured, protecting people from the gore of crucifixion. People don't like to see torture or a reminder of sin. Perhaps here, where there has been war, the reality of pain and death is better understood. Torture, I had learned, was a common occurrence here in Jaffna during the war. Perhaps Jesus understood the struggles of the people.

This little chapel soon became a source of refuge for me. A stolen moment alone. I began running there most days, feeling unobserved in a treasured space not meant for foreign worshipers but open, nonetheless. It was a place for introspection and spiritual grounding.

The coastal area around the chapel had been occupied by the Sinhalese Army during the thirty-year civil war. India was a mere nineteen kilometres across the Indian Ocean, and I had been told that the Sinhalese army feared military support for the Tamil Tigers from among India's large Tamil Nadu population. As a result, the army strategically controlled the coast of Sri Lanka to ensure support did not come from India's Tamil people. The army displaced fishermen and their families from their homes with no compensation and over the years, the homes were shelled and looted, leaving crumbling concrete foundations.

It was sobering to run past these homes on my way to the chapel. I kept imagining the displacement of the people, and the shelling that took place between the Tamil Tigers and the Sinhalese Army. The roofing tiles, the window frames and the flooring had all been taken, stripping the homes of any function or beauty. Weeds grew up through cracked concrete, trees and vines wove themselves in and out of window openings and doorways like serpents—the invasive flora provided the houses with new occupants.

Some days, before entering the church, I waited at a distance, observing a small Tamil boy, about ten years old and barefoot, carrying a red plastic bucket and a mop. Sauntering towards the temple, he bowed, entered the chapel and began sloshing the floor with the soapy water. Smearing the suds in wide circular motions, he soaped the entire surface.

His mopping rinsed off the dust blown in through the open windows. Finally, he pushed the muddy water out through the church entrance and down the two concrete stairs. Soap suds filled the ruts in the red earth by the chapel stairs.

With his chore concluded, he gathered his tools and exited with a small genuflection at Jesus. Scampering off between the abandoned homes, I assumed he readied himself for school.

One day, as I approached, I was surprised to see a Tamil woman clad in a colourful sari, crumpled to the floor either in adoration or beseeching God for some desperate need. She was unaware of my prying eyes in the doorway.

Moved by her posture and devotion, I realised she deserved to be alone with God. I moved away until I saw her leave the chapel. It dawned on me that probably I was not the only one who visited this little chapel in secret.

Only then, when alone, did I tiptoe across the floor to kneel and, once again, I felt I was wearying God with my problems.

Daily, like clockwork, I presented myself to the Cross—each day with a new complaint. I whispered to the Son of God, not the plaster representation, but to the Son himself.

Jesus, I am so lonely. We are hot, we are worried. I am confused, I am so unsure of myself. I don't know how to help. I don't know what to do, help me, show me what you want me to do. I don't know how to proceed, I have nothing to offer, why did you send me here? I was born into privilege. I have never lived through war. How can I possibly be of service?

Blah, blah, blah. I got sick of myself and wondered why God wasn't sick of me too.

Yet, on other days, I was on my knees flushed with gratitude.

Dear God, I am so lucky, thank you for this wonderful opportunity. Thank you for my husband. Thank you for the great friends you have sent. Thank you for allowing me to live in this wonderful warm climate. Thank you for opening my eyes to the beauty of different cultures, for the joy of riding a motorcycle, for the wonder of living by the ocean.

I vacillated between grief and gratitude like a pendulum on a grandfather clock, only logging the extremes and never feeling the mid-point.

I told no one about my morning visits and my inner dialogue with God; they were too private to share, too revealing about my relationship with God and my struggle as a volunteer. I told no one, not even my husband, Bill, that each day, I met with Jesus for support. I felt blessed to have discovered this sanctuary where I took support from the source of strength.

Part One
Becoming a Volunteer

Chapter 1
Unravelling Myself

Kernels of your life's direction are planted, unbeknownst at the time.

In 1986, I was thirty years old, married and the mother of five young children, ranging in age from three to eleven. One evening, after the hectic rounds of rustling up dinner, fighting to get the children to help with dishes, bathing five little bodies, throwing in a load of laundry and even going out to mow the lawn before the rain came, I finally got the children tucked into their beds with a story and a kiss. Silence. Space. Sanctuary.

Back in the kitchen, I filled the kettle and dropped a peppermint tea bag into my cracked mug. As I poured the boiling liquid over the tea bag, it puffed like a marshmallow. I carried my cup to the kitchen nook and shook open the dishevelled daily newspaper.

I was not much of a newspaper reader, but I did like to browse headlines, dream of a new home whilst reading the real estate section, bargain hunt in the want ads, and with morbid curiosity, read the obituaries. I always felt a bit too weary to be interested in the real news. As I browsed, a five-inch by five-inch advertisement caught my eye.

Canadian University Services Overseas (CUSO) was encouraging people to consider volunteering across the globe. CUSO was the Canadian arm of a global Non-Government Organization (NGO) called Volunteer Services Overseas (VSO). CUSO-VSO was recruiting skilled volunteers to work in developing countries to create sustainable change in areas of livelihood/resource management, participation and governance, health, disability, AIDS and HIV and education.

I was inspired, but I wasn't sure I had anything to offer. I had no fancy university degree. I had worked as a waitress and a lifeguard and a swimming instructor. These skills did not seem to be sought after by CUSO. I felt trapped by the lack of opportunity.

Sniffling, I tossed aside the newspaper and began the evening routine of compiling a stack of cheese and lettuce sandwiches for the kids' lunches for the following school day. Falling into bed late that night, I felt exhausted and hopeless. The next morning, after the miracle of sleep, I snipped the article out of the newspaper and placed it into a folder, labelling it 'International Work'. There it sat, forgotten and collecting dust for twenty-three years.

In June of 1990, my marriage unravelled. There was no longer the energy or the will to try and re-wind the yoyo of our relationship. Despite the intense grief, I managed to pull together the strength and organisation required to apply to university. I felt I had an opportunity to take back a lost dream and to be able to provide for my children.

In September of 1990, I entered the University College of the Cariboo (UCC) and learned that the nursing degree program required a full year of science studies. I studied hard, passed the first year successfully, and after my interview, I was offered a seat in the nursing program to begin my second year of university in the fall of 1991.

That's when I got cold feet. Nursing meant shift work, and I had five children to consider. Who would take them to their activities? I also had visions of my kids climbing in through bedroom windows just minutes before I arrived home after a long night shift.

But that wasn't the only reason I was second-guessing my educational decision. Nursing meant precision and accuracy. By then, I knew myself well enough to know that I am a conceptual, abstract thinker, a 'big picture' person. Meticulous attention to detail is not my forte.

I shared my concerns with Butch, the man I was dating at the time. "You know, if the medication dosage for a patient is 7.0 cc, I can see myself drawing up 7.5 cc thinking, 'That is close enough!' I'm liable to kill someone!" I wailed.

"You will have to work at nursing a long time, and it's a torture to work at something you hate or aren't even good at," Butch replied. "You must bite the bullet now if you're going to make a change."

I knew he was right, but my decision to 'bite the bullet' left me with one year of science under my belt and no educational direction. I pored over the university calendar looking for a program of study. Social work seemed intriguing, although I had no idea what a social worker did.

I was fast running out of time to apply for September courses, so I tossed my concerns to the wind. I finished a second year of general arts and applied to the social work program. I felt passionate, excited about the course work and burned with desire to help those less fortunate. I knew that I had found my calling.

My children and I paid a heavy price for my education. Although not a perfectionist, I was tenacious and determined to be the best student and the best Mom at the same time. I was best at neither.

We had precious little money from child support and student loans, and although I was a genius at making money spread to keep the mortgage paid, an old van on the road, the fridge stocked for hungry teenagers, utilities, sporting activities, school supplies, clothing and house repairs, it never seemed like there was enough for all the unexpected expenses that popped up.

We had enough, but what none of us had enough of was time with each other. Too many evenings passed with my nose in a book, leaving precious little time for stories, affection, cuddles, listening, or family time. Each of us was trying to cope, but we were isolated and disengaged.

Four of my children during this time were teenagers, so Mutiny on the Bounty was commonplace as they ganged up against the parental authority to which I clung. I was constantly tired.

Despite these struggles, I thrived at university and in 1994, was nominated valedictorian by the Faculty of Social Work. In my speech, I reminded fellow students that we were **animis opibusque parati**—*prepared in minds and resources*. The night of my graduation, I began dating my now-husband, Bill, a friend from years earlier. I felt I had turned a corner.

A few years later, I was invited by a women's service group to speak at their annual banquet. Their mandate was to encourage and inspire women in difficult circumstances to seek a post-secondary education to become economically independent. I was honoured for the opportunity. I hoped to be a role model that might inspire and cheer other women forward.

Carefully, I scripted my speech, which included some self-disclosure about the grief, the hardships and the struggles I had encountered. As I shared my story with the audience, a loud sob spilled out from me. I did not prepare for, nor expect such an intense emotional response. Tearful, I struggled to compose myself at the podium.

Somehow that sob symbolised a collective grief, centuries old and ancient— a grief that is shared by all men, women and children impacted by divorce. I felt as if every cell in my body contained a memory of my struggle; the memories had embedded themselves into the fibres of my being, stored and dusty, but not forgotten. But by then, I wasn't alone with the remnants of my grief.

In 1996, during one of the worst ice storms in the history of Kamloops, I married Bill. Bill had two children of his own, Rob and Shelley, and he was a joint custodial father at the time. Combined now by marriage, we numbered a family of seven children and two adults, although some of the older children had already left home by the time we married.

We all settled into our new lives. It felt like it held promise.

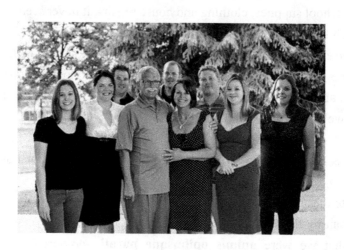

2010: Bill and I and our blended family

Chapter 2
A New Calling

Niggling is the soul's gentle but uncomfortable nudge in the right direction.

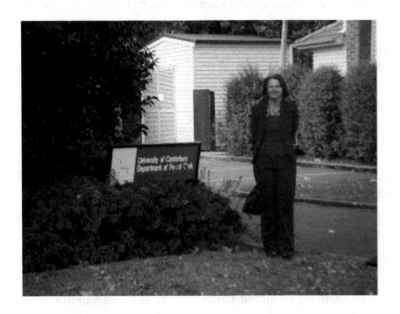

2009: University of Canterbury, New Zealand just after successfully defending my PhD in Social Work

I was born a cradle Catholic. Catholicism is my birth right, passed on to me by my Germanic ancestors and fostered at the knees of my devout father and converted, but even more devout mother. Catholicism was my heritage. Learning to pray the rosary and making my First Communion at age five was like buried treasure leaving me prosperous and affluent in spirtualty.

This affluence saved me the exploration, the indecision, the searching for religion or spirituality besetting so many others. Thus, for me, Catholicism was always a freedom.

My husband, Bill, was an atheist but benevolent to my belief system. When we began dating, he articulated the limitations of his support, "I respect your religious beliefs, but don't ever expect me to become a Catholic."

I didn't have expectations of him to convert. As he respected my beliefs, I respected his atheism. However, to my surprise (and delight), within a couple of years of being married, he began attending mass with me at the small church of Our Lady of Lourdes in Heffley Creek. Somehow, he found something useful in this weekly attendance, and within a few years, after some religious instruction, he was baptised a Catholic. For him, it was a reasoned choice.

Bill and I usually found great solace at mass, but for some unknown reason, an unsettledness came upon us, which manifested itself in church. I began weeping in mass each week. This unsettledness, like an invisible force of destiny, was undefined and nebulous. It seemed to serve no purpose and gave no direction. The inner voice niggled, but it was unintelligible.

There was a hymn written by Daniel L. Schutte in 1981 that I found to be problematic. This hymn was based on Samuel I, Verse Three (1 Samuel 3). In the Old Testament story, Samuel's mother dedicated her infant son to God in thanksgiving for a male child. She placed him in a temple to live and learn from the resident prophet, Eli.

One night, lying on his bed in the temple, Samuel was awakened by a strange voice calling him. "Samuel, Samuel." Samuel scoured the temple, investigating the source of the voice. Finding no one, he returned to his bed. Again, he heard a voice calling him. "Samuel, Samuel."

Again, he searched about but found nobody in the gloom of the temple. By then, Eli had arisen from his bed and searched within the darkened temple until he located Samuel.

"What are you doing, my son?" He asked, peering into the shadows.

Confused, Samuel related his experience of hearing a strange voice that seemed to be calling him as he lay upon his bed. Eli, being an experienced prophet and holy man of God, realised this was the voice of God. He instructed the boy, "Return to your bed and when you again hear the voice calling to you, say, 'Here I am, Lord, I'm listening'."

This story not only haunted me, but Bill as well. Samuel became a symbol for our search. Like Samuel, we were hearing a voice calling but its requests were shapeless, fluid. Like Samuel, we were calling out, "Here I am. I will go Lord if you lead me." But where were we being led?

I began going to daily morning mass to find some direction, some purpose. Daily sermons delivered by our priest spoke to me, questioning, prodding and provoking me.

"What is your purpose?" The priest asked one week.

"What is God's plan for you?" He inquired the following week.

"What are you doing with your life?" He pressed the week after.

"How can you give back?" He persisted.

On and on, it went. On many Sundays, hot, silent tears slid down my cheek. I stifled the sniffling and wiped my snotty nose against my sleeve and discretely smeared the salty tears. Later in the car, often still parked in the church parking lot, Bill and I disclosed our mutual feelings. We seemed driven to do something in gratitude for our abundant life but had no idea what to do. It was disquieting.

Soon, a persistent form was bubbling up inside me, almost imperceptible. However, all my being resisted what was being suggested. "You need your PhD." I had completed my master's degree in 2002.

It exemplified a level of education far above any dreams I had held for myself. I yearned for nothing further. "No," I told God. "I am tired."

I told Him I needed stability. More than anything, I needed personal space and free time. I needed to work at my marriage, focus on my career and enjoy the crop of grandchildren sprouting from the marriages of my children. Yet, this haunting urge continued.

"Go and get your PhD," He encouraged. "I will give you the energy," God said, infusing hope.

"I don't have the money for a post-graduate program. I have just spent thousands on my master's degree," I pleaded with Him to understand. I dug in my heels. This was not what I had in mind. I thought he was going to send me on a special mission of great importance. I was going to be the next Nelson Mandela or Mother Teresa.

"You will need your PhD. Don't worry about the money."

"What about my kids, God?" I sputtered. "Haven't they been through enough already with my nose in a book all the time?"

"Wendy, they will be fine. I will take care of them."

The more I protested, the tauter the tension became. This debate with God seesawed back and forth for almost two years until finally, my resistance was crumbling, and I started to feel a niggling desire to study for the PhD. In 2005, I found myself traversing PhD programs in social work.

I found an intriguing program and applied to the University of Canterbury in New Zealand. That same year, my research proposal was accepted. I was to be a distance student with residency requirements. My post-graduate studies commenced.

I chose New Zealand because I know my husband. The travel bug consumes Bill. He was thrilled to accompany me to New Zealand, and he willingly allocated our funds towards tuition. I had set up the lack of money as my primary barrier to study, but with Bill's support, this barrier collapsed. Other barriers crashed as well.

By some great stroke of luck and good timing, the New Zealand Ministry of Education had instituted a program to attract PhD students from abroad, and as a result, I qualified for domestic student rates rather than the exorbitant foreign student fees. My tuition was cheaper than my undergraduate program had been!

As for the children, they were launching as well. In university themselves or working full time, they no longer needed me in the same capacity. The final protest about tiredness was shushed and my physical health surged with new energy.

Throughout 2005, I worked full time at the hospital in Kamloops, and in the quiet of dawn and in the late hours of the night, I began structuring the PhD research. I researched and read, poring over, marking up and making notes on peer-reviewed medical and social work journals at coffee breaks, lunch breaks and between clients. By 2007, the double duty of full-time work and full-time research amplified, leaving me a bit threadbare. Deciding I needed more free time, I shifted gears.

I sat and passed a clinical therapy exam. With this new designation as a registered clinical social worker, I left my full-time social work practice in psychiatry at the hospital. Starting a private practice in a local psychiatrist's office afforded me a good income, fewer hours and the blessed flexibility to study, research and vacation. Another barrier was removed.

On 9 April 2009, I walked across the graceful campus of the University of Canterbury in Christchurch, New Zealand. I wore a new brown suit and a red blouse. I had my hair cut and coloured that morning. I needed to look competent, polished and learned.

I meandered past the flowering Kowhai and hairy orchids and ducked under golden tree ferns. I sniffed the air as I walked past the lovely coffee shops where I used to drink long blacks on my breaks from thesis writing. I said goodbye to the lemon tree that rustled against my office window and ripened its sour yellow fruit I used for my tea each day.

That day, I defended my doctoral thesis, entitled *Insight into Insight: a study on understanding schizophrenia*. After defending my thesis to a panel of examiners, my professor, Dr Kate van Heugten, ushered me back through the lush flowering courtyard and into the staff room to wait while the examiners deliberated. Twenty terse minutes later, Kate and I reversed our steps. As we stepped into the small examination room, the lead examiner stood and bowed. "Congratulations, Dr Nordick."

Out of my mouth blurted one of those strange sobs. My inner critic chided, "Not very professional, Dr Nordick." I dashed the tears from my eyes as I shook hands, accepting congratulations from the examiners. My soul rejoiced, singing its own alleluia.

I received another gift that day. Throughout the entire four and a half years of my studies, my professor Kate, was a kind yet objective professional. The evening of my defence, she offered to take Bill and me to a local Indian restaurant to celebrate. Over red wine and crispy onion bhajis, Kate surprised us with her warmth, humour and honesty.

That night, with her dark eyes peering into my soul, she raised her wine glass, toasting, "Wendy, it has always been your destiny to become a doctor. It can never be taken away from you. It is who you are, Dr Nordick." I sighed in contentment. Onion bhajis never tasted better.

Back in Canada, I continued daily mass. Amidst the slow shuffling of soled feet up to communion, the priest holding the white Host high while whispering, "The Body of Christ," and the responding hushed amens, the nagging continued.

What am I supposed to do?

What do you want from me?

What is my purpose?

However, God was silent. I felt tortured and so did Bill. Bill by now was fully retired and getting antsier by the day to 'get going' with his life. But he had no idea what 'getting going' was supposed to look like. He only knew he wanted to travel.

We both took an English as a Second Language (ESL) course but teaching ESL didn't seem to be our calling. Moaning and groaning, we shook our fist at God, "What are we supposed to do?"

One ordinary day at my private practice office, I was purging my file cabinet of old papers. Weeding down into the last drawer, I stumbled upon that sloppily labelled folder marked 'International Work'. Blowing off the dust, I opened the yellowed folder. Out tumbled the brittle newspaper ad about CUSO, the advertisement I had clipped so many years earlier.

Reading that faded ad again, I knew I was different. I had a marketable skill born from God's nagging to get it, and I was no longer a mother of young children. I dashed to my computer.

Google sizzled as I snooped through CUSO's colourful and interactive website. Reading testimonials and stories of 'returned volunteers', my excitement grew. I clicked open the Volunteer Application. I completed it and pressed send. That afternoon, I returned home from work and announced, "Bill, I applied to CUSO today."

"You did?" He shrieked. "Then so will I," he said, scrambling to his computer. Bill had his own desire to volunteer. He had first heard of CUSO in the 1960s while studying his undergraduate degree at the University of British Columbia.

I hovered over his shoulder as he pecked at the keyboard. He was grinning. We have finally found our calling and the nagging in church ceased.

Chapter 3
Preparing for Change

Prepare, prepare and there will be less repair.

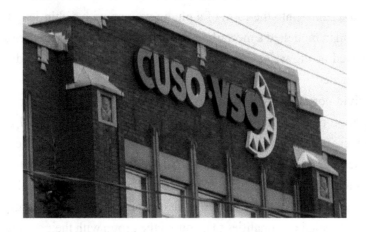

2009: CUSO-VSO office in Ottawa

One morning in May 2009, the phone rang. Busy washing up breakfast dishes, I answered the kitchen wall phone, soap bubbles dripping from my hands onto the green tiled floor. It was Kathryn from CUSO. Our applications had already been processed, and she was offering us an interview.

Delighted, we booked the date and time, and a few days later, Kathryn interviewed us by telephone. For an hour, we chatted about our motives and desire to work for CUSO. We highlighted our education whilst expressing our willingness to serve in any suitable capacity. Kathryn made us feel comfortable.

We must have passed the mystery job selection criteria as within a month, we were speeding down the Coquihalla superhighway towards Vancouver, British Columbia. We had been invited to attend a group interview. The morning of the interview, we hustled down Burrard Street from our hotel to the local YM/YWCA building where CUSO had rented space for the interview process.

Besides Bill and me, a dozen other candidates milled nervously about the lobby. We eyed our competitors with some wariness.

As we introduced ourselves, we learned that candidates were not only Canadians, but Americans as well. CUSO is the Canadian counterpart of the international organisation, Volunteer Services Overseas (VSO), and they had amalgamated into an international group called CUSO International, or CUSO-VSO.

The interview took a full day. It was unlike any job evaluation we had ever attended. To start with, we were asked to draw self-portraits. In red ink, I dragged the felt marker lines into the form of a plump woman with a chin-length bob.

This woman modelled a mortarboard with tassel, but also, she wore a kitchen apron cinched at the waist. She was my domestic self and my academic self. They had melded.

The vivid portrait drawn from my subconscious was visceral for me. I saw the integration of my different roles; I was not segmented nor was I polarised. My roles were not compartmentalised but holistic—one did not negate the other. Tears welled as I explained my portrait to my fellow candidates. My hands were shaking, and I was embarrassed by the emotional response to this realisation.

We played games in the interview which required teamwork and discussion. The games revealed personalities that soured the group with their aggression and the group lost respect for those who acquiesced. They also revealed the team players and the problem solvers, and yet somehow, the puzzles were only solved with group input.

I recognised that while not a strong leader, I was willing to take more risk than others and think outside the box. Bill emerged as the voice of reason.

At the end of the day, some of us dashed to a nearby Irish pub for a necessary debriefing and to quell the pent-up anxiety with a cold beer. The green shamrocks that festooned the walls of the pub animated us as we examined, rehashed, discussed and admired the genius of the unique process we had just experienced. We were no longer rivals but colleagues.

We drove home from Vancouver wondering if we had a future with CUSO. Did they like us? Did they think we had the 'right' criteria? The other candidates demonstrated intelligence, were fun, extroverted and seemed like-minded, but we had no idea what qualities were going to snare those coveted international positions.

Lacking confidence, we judged ourselves by the brilliance of the others, felt dumb and too mundane to be selected. For two weeks, we sat on pins and needles, vacillating between defence mechanisms reflecting our fear of rejection. 'I don't care if we don't get accepted' and 'What the hell are they looking for anyway?' We felt stressed, our self-esteem ruffled with the wait.

Then the phone rang. CUSO invited us to a second telephone interview. We began to feel superior and special that we were moving upward through the selection process. As we sat at our kitchen table speaking with the CUSO recruiter on the phone, we gazed out our large kitchen window. A tawny mule deer meandered into our park-like back yard searching for my pink sedums they loved nibbling upon. We couldn't help but wonder if the deer was a sign of our dreams coming true.

A week later, we received a phone call from a CUSO staff member, "You and Bill have both been accepted as volunteers. How soon can you come to Ottawa for the 'Preparing for Change' course?"

"We're happy to go as soon as possible."

"That's great!" the woman on the phone replied. "The next course is in September."

"We will be there," we decided. CUSO booked our flights and hotel.

The anticipation was delicious. Our excitement rode high for the remainder of the summer. In September, as the sun thinned and the trees in the yard were changing their robes from green to gold, we boarded a jet for Ottawa, Ontario. The next morning, after polishing off a hearty bowl of oatmeal with fresh cream and blueberries in the small hotel cafeteria, we set off on foot for the CUSO office.

The air was crisp and cool, our breath visible as we puffed along. Coloured maple leaves left their twiggy toggles and drifted down about us as we treaded along sidewalks covered in the slippery red, yellow and orange of the already fallen. We trundled over a bridge into a somewhat run-down industrial section, a mixed neighbourhood of older, solid, middle-class homes and modest office buildings. We turned left onto Eccles Street and caught sight of a four-story, red-bricked building with a sign at the very top that read 'CUSO-VSO'.

The unassuming exterior disguised the vibrancy within the building. Bright posters and photographs of volunteers working in different countries adorned the walls, their variety giving perspective to the mandate and scope of the organisation. We gaped at the pictures adorning the ever-crowding lobby waiting for the receptionist to appear. Others were milling about, doing the same.

As if a tiny bell had been tinkled suggesting a start, office doors flew open, and staff began emerging from all corners of the building. The skin of the staff members reflected a bright spectrum of colour, white alabaster to inky black with hues and shades of mocha in between. They greeted us in English, but with vowel sounds elongated or alternatively clipped, with different emphases on syllables, voices deep in timber or pitched in singsong.

"Huulloo!"

"Wheelcommm!"

"Noiss to meet you!"

A tall black woman wore a headscarf over cornrow braids. Another regal woman was wrapped in a royal blue shawl. Several strands of large, beaded necklaces adorned another woman's long slim neck. A bald man with a shiny black head had donned an African tunic woven with geometric shapes in amber, orange and black.

I was overwhelmed. The rich colours and vibrancy of the atmosphere teleported me into another world. Although, I was in Ottawa, I was a visible, drab minority in my North American costume of blue jeans and white T-shirt. This display of diversity was preparing us for the cultural experience that lay ahead.

We were directed into a large open room adjacent to the lobby. As we mingled, greeting one another, other volunteers asked us, "To which country have you been assigned?" It became clear that most of the volunteers already had assignments. Many were flying directly from the training to their new country.

Abashed, we stopped feeling like we were somehow superior or special. We were way behind everyone else. Our spirits drooped.

The weekend began with clever icebreaker games forcing us to interact. We met our volunteer colleagues. Charles and Shawna were teachers, Terry was an artist, Dudley was a businessman and Mary and Monique were accountants. Chris was a development worker. Jenny was a lawyer.

The occupational mix was suggestive of the variety of placements CUSO offered. The variety of people in the room also revealed that international volunteering holds a universal appeal.

Our shyness slid away and was replaced by laughter and a growing familiarity. Videos depicting other volunteers' experiences awed us and left us doubting our own abilities. Lectures on social and political orientations gave us the knowledge and skills needed to learn more about the country we might be assigned. Discussions and think tanks were useful in preparing us for a cultural work experience where values, norms, beliefs and practices differed from our own.

We played a banking game, which came with no instructions. We were assigned roles such as villager, farmer, woman, person of lower caste and a rich businessman. A CUSO staff member was the banker.

We soon learned that women could not meet with the banker without a male escort. A farmer was not allowed into the bank unless invited by an existing member of the bank and only those assigned power, such as the rich businessman, had access to the banking institution and its lending policies.

We learned the rules of the pseudo culture through trial and error and figured out how to acknowledge, wield, access, or circumvent power to obtain cash. People with a lower cultural status were never able to access money, which forced them to cajole, wield and distort the truth. It demonstrated the complexity of business in some countries.

Women, the lower caste and the poor, shouldered social exclusion and financial inequality. Power, privilege and corruption were the regime of patriarchy and the banker. These lessons proved useful.

These games and role-plays forced us to manage conflict, face corruption and reflect on personal safety. Situations were designed to challenge us to think about how we might accomplish sustainable development when the rules and norms differed from our own worldview.

In one scenario, Bill was assigned a role as a village chieftain. He was handed a dishtowel as a piece of costume, which he tied around his head. He looked exotic with his striped headscarf and big blonde moustache. His task was to conduct a meeting between volunteers and his villagers.

Female villagers were not allowed to speak to him, except through their husbands or a male family member. When a female volunteer tried to approach him, he wrinkled his nose, turning his back in affront. The experience resulted in a hilarious role-play but with dark undertones of the inequality and treatment of women in some cultures. The role-plays planted seeds of angst at the challenges ahead.

This same weekend, we were each assigned a CUSO advisor. Our advisor, as it turned out, was Kathryn, the same CUSO staff member involved in our original telephone interview. Personable and warm, she called us from the ongoing sessions and led us to her cosy office.

This informal discussion gave her perspective on the ideas we had formulated about where we might like to go and what we might like to do within the six categories of service provision of CUSO. She assessed our needs and desires, and based on these desires, our occupations and our experience, explored options for placement.

In this meeting, our hopes were dashed. We had hoped for an opportunity to work in Mexico, South or Central America, but we were not going to be assigned a Spanish-speaking country. Kathryn explained that language was a critical barrier in development work and most of the positions in Spanish language regions were assigned to those with some fluency in Spanish.

Although Bill and I had taken a few informal Spanish courses over the years, we had forgotten most of what we had learned. We knew we couldn't fake fluency.

Kathryn advised us that there were several positions she was considering for us, but she had to formalise some arrangements and determine placement dates. She cautioned that it could take time to place a volunteer, particularly two volunteers in the same location, each with different skill sets (me in social work/mental health and Bill in legal/ governance areas). Patience was advised.

She explained that a good fit was critical to sustainable development and the satisfaction of the placement, both from the volunteer's as well as the placement organisation's perspective.

However, she put forth some initial positions for us to consider. The first position offered was for Bill. The position was in Kingston, Jamaica, training Supreme Court justices. As Bill had served as a Provincial Court judge in British Columbia for over twenty-six years, this position appeared to be a perfect fit for his skill set.

However, we longed for a country where English was not the first language. We fancied the opportunity of the language challenge, naïve to the difficulty of learning and working in a second language. Besides, we both knew that Jamaica had one of the highest murder rates in the world, which was a huge deterrent for us.

The second position Kathryn asked us to consider was a social work position in Mongolia. Mongolia didn't thrill us either. We had imagined ourselves volunteering in a tropical climate—it was part of the dream. Huddling up to a tiny stove in a yurt of animal hide and wearing fur and wool to stay warm wasn't part of our adventure list. We didn't endure cold weather well anymore.

Then, Kathryn sat forward and whispered, as if in a clandestine rendezvous, "I'm very excited about another possibility for you, Wendy. The war in Sri Lanka is now over and we believe we can get a social worker to Jaffna to work with people affected by the war. This is a top priority for us. Would you be willing to wait and see if this goes through?"

She explained that CUSO-VSO had been trying to place a social worker in Jaffna for several years, but due to the thirty-year civil war, the visa restrictions made placing a social worker in the region impossible. We agreed to wait.

"Oh, there's one more thing," she said. "As you know, we expect a two-year commitment from all our volunteers."

"What?" I gaped at her. "I thought the placements were three to six months."

Kathryn shook her head. "No, Wendy, there are twelve to eighteen-month-long placements, but this placement will be two years."

Two years? We were stunned and dismayed. But we were in too deep to back out. We agreed to the two-year commitment, wondering how we would break this news to our kids and my parents.

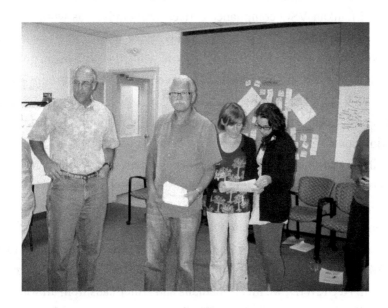

2009: Preparing for Change Course in Ottawa with other outgoing volunteers

Chapter 4
New Skills, New Friends

The more unique and special we think we are, the more likely we are to learn
how unique and special others really are.

We travelled home from the PFC weekend unsure of our future. Thrill coursed through us as we dissected the possibilities of each of the positions offered. We scoured world maps to locate the geographical location of Sri Lanka, Mongolia and Jamaica.

The local public library and second-hand bookstores provided us with additional reading materials. We explored the political situation, the economics, the environment and the intricacies of how society overlapped culture.

While we waited to hear from Kathryn, we continued to hold out hope for the Sri Lankan position as it held the most intrigue. From time to time, a call or email came from her updating us on the visa situation in Sri Lanka. We were told that the Sri Lankan VSO compliance officer, Manchula, was working with the visa office in Colombo.

The situation was deemed 'tricky' because while the Sri Lankan government wanted NGO support and funding, it was nervous about NGO scrutiny inside the country. VSO believed this nervousness was due to possible and subsequent demands or condemnation from the international community regarding human rights violations.

Finally, Kathryn called with no small excitement in her voice. "Manchula is fairly certain we will be obtaining visas for the both of you for Sri Lanka!" she said. "So, you are invited to attend the 'Skills and Knowledge for Working in Development' (SKWID) course in Ottawa in October."

A hearty cheer escaped us. In October 2009, we flew back to Ottawa to attend the SKWID course, a mandatory for preparing volunteers for an international assignment. At SKWID, we met Canadians and Americans from all walks of life and ages. We learned more about CUSO as an organisation. Dr Mark Wise,

32

tropical disease specialist and author of the book, *Travel Health Guide,* gave us tips for health when working abroad.

Our judgments and biases about other cultures were once again exposed through role-play and games. This time, one of the games involved an NGO assisting villagers to build a bridge across the river that had been diverted upstream and now divided a village. Volunteers were assigned as engineers and none of the engineers spoke Tsmiligee, the fictional language of the village, so signing and body language were used to communicate.

The engineers waved and gestured and shouted in English when they were not understood. Guttural responses along with tongue clicks accompanied the 'villagers' gestures as they explained their needs for the bridge and how and where it needed to be constructed. It was interesting to see how intercultural communication can take place without language.

CUSO staff drilled home the importance of setting up measures and evaluation tools to quantify results. We learned about the dichotomy between volunteer expectations of the experience and the reality. They drew a trough graph depicting the process of enculturation.

During the honeymoon period of moving to a country everything seems wonderful, new and exciting, but as time goes on, the flaws of the country become more apparent. Thus, feelings of disappointment, loneliness and anger might arise. The volunteer is in the trough. Then, as the volunteer makes shifts and adjustments to the reality of the situation, they begin to climb out of the trough.

CUSO staff also explained the potential difficulties with re-integration when the volunteer returns home. Bill and I were pretty sure we could handle the culture shock and wouldn't be sliding into a trough. We were tough.

About thirty volunteers attended the SKWID course and most of them had their marching orders to their respective countries. Almost all were in various stages of selling cars and furniture and either selling or renting their homes, as we were planning to do.

Michelle, an outgoing and forthright French-Canadian woman, about fifty years of age, was assigned to Burkina Faso for eighteen months. She was leaving from the training weekend to the airport for her flight out. She had already arranged a leave of absence from her accounting firm, sold her home in downtown Montreal and sold her car. She expressed her trepidation about what she was about to do, how stressful it had been getting all her ducks in a row to leave, and yet how excited she was to go.

Charles, an affable man from the Windsor area, was heading into Nigeria for two years. A retired high school principal, his venture abroad as a volunteer was fulfilling a life's dream to go back to his roots in Africa and 'give back'. He was to assist in the curriculum and staff development of high school programming and teachers.

His wife of twenty-five years was not accompanying him, yet she did plan to visit him. We admired the strength of his marriage to leave his spouse behind for two years. Bill and I were not sure we could make that same commitment.

We met Wendy and her husband, Greg, who were experienced volunteers. Twenty-some years ago, they packed up all their pre-school aged children and set off to Papua, New Guinea where they volunteered for VSO for two years. Their experience was so rich that they were back for another experience now that their children were all adults.

We admired their sense of adventure and their unique experiences as we stared at their photographs of thin, black, scantily clad aboriginal people holding spears and sporting golden collars. They stood with painted white stripes gracing their cheeks and tenderly held this couple's tiny, blond child in their arms.

The week of SKWID bonded us together. Common to all of us was the stress of taking care of all the details involved in a move across an ocean; the excitement and adventure of travel; the ambivalence about how to be effective as a development worker; the surprise from friends and family in response to us doing something out of the ordinary, and the uncertainty of the future. We discussed how to leave loved ones so they didn't feel abandoned. I shared my guilt of leaving behind aging parents and young grandchildren.

The last evening of training, we crowded into a Sri Lankan restaurant near the VSO office. Smelling of curry and spice, the tiny restaurant was decorated with Ganesh and other Hindu deities. Buddha sat in a corner, holding court. We relied on CUSO staff to order for us.

We ate chickpea curry and potato curry mixed with spicy sambal and egg hoppers. We had no idea such foods existed. One man ordered a dosai. A white crepe-like roll arrived, twice the size of his plate. Another ordered a feast of string hoppers, a nest of noodles resembling a twisted ball of snakes in a snake den. The exotic foods were delicious, whetting our appetite for more.

Hugging each other goodbye, we swapped email addresses, wished each other safe travels and after promising to stay in touch, we gave one last wistful wave to each other. Our new friends all boarded jets to far-flung countries. Bill and I boarded an Air Canada jet and flew back home to Kamloops. We were still grounded for lack of a work visa.

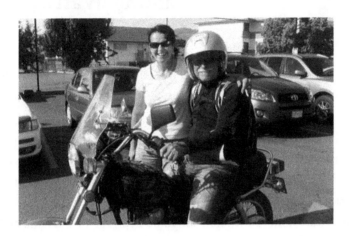

Bill and I taking our motorbike training prior to departure

Chapter 5
The Never-Ending Wait

Waiting does not require patience. Waiting is the careful honouring of
God's will and time for us.

We returned home from SKWID with sugarplums dancing in our heads. Nervous energy drove us yet immobilised us. We continued to fuss. All our seven children were doing well. They were robust, had great jobs and great parenting skills. However, we stewed.

Our little grandchildren would soon to be deprived of grandma and grandpa days. What about my parents? What about my private practice? I loved my family therapy practice and I wrung my hands at the idea of closing my office and the potential of not having work when I returned.

We also fretted about renting our home after hearing stories of tenants trashing rental homes. Would our home suffer a similar fate?

This hive of worries buzzed around us. However, determination to proceed prevailed. Later that month, Kathryn called, her voice elevated in excitement, "I spoke with the VSO Colombo office today. Manchula is convinced a visa clearance is pending. I am going to go ahead and book your flights to Colombo." Our leaving date was scheduled for 5 January 2010. The time had come. I closed my cosy private practice office.

We packed and sorted. Sitting crossed legged in front of boxes in the basement, we separated the essentials from the junk we'd been collecting over the past fifteen years. Yes, quilts were necessary. No, cracked dishes were not. We sorted pictures and keepsakes, a slow-going, thoughtful process.

Each item flooded us with memories that we shared with one another. What was not necessary, sentimental or valuable was shoved into a box and Bill, shaking his head at this accumulation of what he called 'stuff', whisked off another load to the nearby thrift shop. We posted rental ads listing our house and ski condo on Kijiji.

There was a mass of 'Bon Voyage' parties and Christmas parties with our family and friends. They seemed even more dusted with Christmas magic. We planned to stay with my parents for the remaining few days before we were scheduled to leave. Then, the unexpected happened.

On 28 December, we received a call from Kathryn telling us that the Sri Lankan government reneged on a work visa for us. CUSO cancelled our flights and rebooked us for April. Disappointment prevailed before fear crept in.

There we were. No jobs. No house. What were we going to do?

Devastated, we decided to lick our wounds and wait for the visa in Mexico. We slung on our loaded, yellow Asolo backpacks and boarded a plane to Mexico City. We bussed all the way to Veracruz, while munching on soggy lunches provided by the coach crew.

In Veracruz, a small hurricane had twisted through, littering the streets with broken palm and chunks of sheet metal. Bill, overcome by the heavy rain and angry with the weather gods, declared, "Hang the cost. We are flying back to the Pacific side where it is warm." Several hundred dollars poorer and eight hours later, we were back in tropical heat. We toured Puerto Vallarta, Guadalajara and Mazatlan.

Our modest hotel in Mazatlan was situated along the Malecon between El Centro and the reams of luxury hotels that towered along the beach of the Pacific Ocean. One afternoon, we lounged around the pool deck on white chaise lounges, soaking up the sun's heat and pretending not to worry about our visa situation. I was just about to feel relaxed when I heard shots. I sat bolt upright.

"Bill, I think that was a gunshot," I gasped as I spun my head towards the sound. There was screaming and more shots were fired in rapid succession. A horde of people from the hotel came fleeing out to the pool. I flew off my chaise and bolted into a nearby pool shed.

I ducked under a peeling sandwich board advertising a lunch special. My eyes darted about the pool area. I witnessed Bill leaping the corner of the pool and pasting himself to the rough cement deck.

After the shots stopped, Bill tiptoed over to me and whispered, "I'm going to the lobby to investigate." From my hiding place, I could see that others were starting to move back into the hotel. I continued to cower under the sandwich board until Bill returned, his face ashen, "There is a man with a bullet in his head lying on the street."

I untangled myself and crept into the shiny, white-tiled lobby with Bill. A young man, wearing an orange T-shirt and blue jean shorts, white sport socks and black shoes lay face up on the street, arms and legs splayed. He was dead. Bright red blood seeped from the single bullet wound in the middle of his forehead and turned to rust as it met the sizzling pavement. A crowd of shocked onlookers was gathering along with a chorus of sirens from arriving police vehicles and the ambulance.

Shaken, Bill and I climbed the stairs to our hotel room on the fifth floor and watched the beehive of activity taking place on the street below. Uniformed policia and non-uniformed crime investigators swarmed the road, consulting with one another. They dragged measuring tapes from their cruisers and began measuring distances between the body and the curb.

In chalk, they drew an outline around the sprawled body whose flesh now cooked in the heat. They searched and collected shell casings, dropping them into plastic baggies. They scribbled in notebooks they dug from their pockets. The man in the orange T-shirt lay there, his head no longer bleeding.

Just minutes earlier, he had been going about his daily business but now lay inert, unaware of the investigation, the crowd and the heat. The next morning, the newspapers cried out, "Violencia." Five assassinations had occurred that day in the city, all drug gang related.

That very night, we awakened to another street scene. An eight-piece band that wielded a flatulent tuba, a full base drum set complete with cymbals, an electric guitar and a bugle began playing outside the hotel from the back of a white pick-up truck at full volume. While they played, an inebriated Mexican man in a white shirt and black pants belted out Spanish love songs. We just shook our heads and chuckled. In his underwear, Bill shouted his joy into the night from our deck, "Viva Mexico."

It was late March now and our new departure date was looming. It was time to go home, back to Canada. Then, it happened. VSO in Colombo informed us that we were again denied a work visa to Jaffna. Our flight was once again re-booked, this time for September.

This gave us some time to get our motorbike license. The program office in Sri Lanka required that I be 'comfortable' on a motorbike as it was going to be necessary to navigate a 63-kilometre loop between hospitals, mental health offices and the universities. In the training, we chugged around bright orange pylon cones laid out in figure eight patterns by our Polish driving instructor, John.

Bill had reasonable control over his bike, but my bike came out of the shoot snorting like a bucking bronco and speeding towards the concrete wall at the far end of the parking lot. Terrified, I was convinced I was going to be dead before leaving the parking lot. I replayed my mantra, *I am smart, I can learn. I am smart, I can learn.*

I had to pass this course. As I bucked around the parking lot, I began to pray. "Dear God, please don't let me kill myself on the motorcycle. Please don't let me kill someone. Give me coordination to pass the skills test."

God didn't answer my prayers. I failed the examination, which provoked even more anxiety about the re-exam. Bill and I decided I needed more practice, so I bought a small Honda 250 cc. Each day, I squished my hairdo under the giant crash helmet, donned my blue jeans, leather jacket and leather boots, pulled on my leather riding gloves, swung my leg over the seat and kicked back the kickstand.

Straddling the bike, I reviewed the basics. Brake and clutch depressed. Right. Press the starter button. Right. Signal and ease off the brake while letting out the clutch. Stalling was a ritual as was failing to flick off my turn signal.

I cruised quiet neighbourhoods, hoping some child didn't dash into the street, hoping the corners were well rounded and hoping nobody was behind me when I had to stop. I was terrified. But I did learn, and I did become competent. When I passed the re-exam, my examiner told me that I had always been a good driver with excellent balance, but I had lacked confidence. I was now confident.

During our wait, we enjoyed a summer socialising with family and friends. In September 2010, we were notified the visa was not granted again, so we shuffled our few belongings into our car and moved into our cabin at Kamloops Lake. I had never stayed at the lake in the late fall. I found it hushed and beautiful.

Over time, the trees morphed their summer green to the red and yellow cloak of fall and then shed their clothing altogether onto the pebbled beach. They stood naked and unprotected before winter's cutting wind. Deer fed on the beach at night and Rocky Mountain sheep with enormous, curled horns began flocking and rutting in large groups.

Our new departure date was now scheduled for 26 October. Bill believed that we would really depart this time, but I pulled up on lap robe of scepticism as protection. We had had so many disappointments. As before, we said our goodbyes to everyone. George Elliot in her outstanding book, *Middlemarch*, hit a little too close to home when she wrote the following: "It is certainly trying to a man's dignity to reappear when he is not expected to do so: a first farewell has pathos in it, but to come back for a second, lends an opening to comedy..." We were beginning to feel foolish.

A few days later, an email arrived from CUSO-VSO:

Dear Wendy,

I am writing to give an update on the visa situation here in Sri Lanka. You will be aware that for a long time there has been a complex process for obtaining visas for volunteers and staff. Over the past three months the government has been instituting a new process for visas, which involves obtaining security clearance before the granting of visas.

Previously, visas were granted and the clearance applied for after arrival. Unfortunately, this new process is proving to be a lengthy one.

We currently have eleven people at various stages of the entry visa process. Although your papers are in the process, we have been informed that it is likely to take another four to five weeks before security clearance is granted. This means that it will not be possible to keep to the planned entry date of 26 October. Rather than setting another date that might have to change again, we will contact you as soon as we have the approved security clearance.

I realise that this news will be disappointing and very frustrating. Please be assured that we are doing all we can on this end to meet the government requirements and allow you to start the important work of your placements.

Sincerely,
Kathryn
VSO

We were stuck between a rock and a hard place. We wanted to volunteer, but we couldn't get a visa. We wanted our home back but had signed a two-year lease agreement that prevented us from breaking a contract. We wanted to secure a temporary home, but this meant yet another move for us.

Our situation distressed our friends and family. Joan and Jim offered us the guesthouse on their property. My sister, Linda, through tears, offered a bedroom in their home. Chris and Mary offered us an opportunity to house-sit for them while they were in Australia.

My dad just shook his head in disbelief and concern. My daughter, Lisa, yelled at us to stop the Sri Lanka process and look elsewhere for volunteer work. So, I set the record straight with our family and friends in this missive from my blog.

Just to be clear; we do have control over this process. We can stop this volunteer process with CUSO whenever we want. Our current chaos is not meant to create chaos for any of our family, friends or readers.

All we ask is that you just sit back and enjoy (vicariously) our ride. Just because this process feels like a ride into Hades, it doesn't mean we want to get off the trolley. We enjoy the thrill that comes when the cart goes downhill.

Back at the lake, we bundled in warm fleeces, reading our Kindles by camp firelight. Dawn found us sipping dark hot Costa Rican coffee and blowing steam across the coffee mugs into the cooling fall air. We loved watching the Canadian geese flock and listening to them honking their marching orders to one another as they prepared for their flight.

What could be more peaceful and renewing? It was romantic. We felt liberated.

As lovely as the lake was by day, the cabin became less than friendly by night, with cold fingering in first to our lower backs and then out to the extremities, our breath visible in the single propane lamplight. With no external source of heat to take off the unpleasant chill, we crawled into bed earlier and earlier in the evening to keep warm, snuggling and wrapping up into each other to preserve body heat.

Soon, daytime warmth thinned to frost and we were miserable. With our tails between our legs, we loaded our meagre belongings back into the car, covered the furniture, scrubbed up the cabin and locked the door for winter. We drove up the hill saying goodbye to the bleak lake. In town, we rented an older, tiny but cosy basement suite to sit out the year.

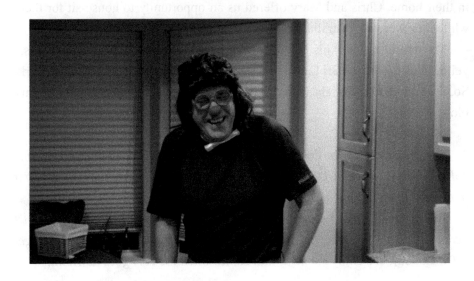

Our friend, Ron Albinson, at a Halloween Bon Voyage party for us (2009)

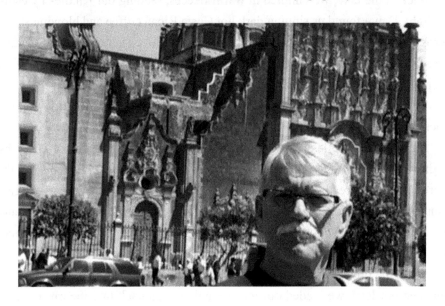

March 2010: Bill in front of Cathedral in Mexico City:
Still waiting for Visa clearance

Chapter 6
Re-Evaluating Our Decision

Knowing exactly what you want and when you want it, is like a stew without
spice. There always seems to be a missing ingredient.

By this time, we felt a sinking realisation that we might never get to Sri Lanka.
We telephoned Kathryn and explained that we were still being patient but made
it clear that we needed employment or needed our homes back if the Sri Lanka
plans fell through. We proposed to CUSO that they secure us an alternative
placement, otherwise we were removing ourselves from the process. CUSO
apologised for the inconvenience, although we knew it was also outside of their
control.

The civil war in Sri Lanka was an ethnic and religious war for equality. Sri
Lanka had been colonised by European powers since the 16th century. After
1815, the British ruled the entire nation until political independence was granted
in 1948. Sri Lanka became a sovereign state after 1972.

The Sinhalese make up about 74% of the population of Sri Lanka. The Sri
Lankan Tamils make up 12.6% and Indian Tamils make up about 5.5% of the
population, while the other 7.1% is made up of Moors and Burghers. The country
is divided not only by race but also by religion.

A 20 Gallup poll indicated that Sri Lanka is the most religious country in the
world with 99% of the people reporting religion as very important to their life.
The 2011 census reported that the Sinhalese Buddhist make up 70.1% of the
population, Hindi (Tamil) make up 2.6% of the population, 9.7% are Muslims
while 6.2% are Roman Catholic and 1.4% are listed as other.

The Sri Lankan Tamils are the largest minority population, but when it comes
to voting in parliament, they are underrepresented and hold no real political
power. Even though Tamil people had lobbied the Sinhalese-controlled
government, requesting extra seats in parliament, the 1972 Constitution declared

Sri Lanka a republic with Buddhism as the state religion and Sinhala as the official language.

As Gordon Weiss (2012), the author of *The Cage: The Fight for Sri Lanka and the Last Days of the Tamil Tigers* pointed out, "the chauvinistic constitution of 1972 sent a message to millions of Tamil citizens that their expectations in Sri Lanka could be comprised of nothing more than an entrenched status as second-class citizens" (p. 48). This is what led to the formation of the Liberation Tigers of Tamil Eelam (LTTE) and the move towards a fight to create an independent Tamil state (Tamil Eelam) in the north and the east of the island where the Tamil people are concentrated.

The civil war started in 1983 and ended in 2009, when the government overthrew the rebel LTTE, but the United Nations Secretary-General, Ban Ki-moon, called for an international panel to advise him on the suspected war crimes in Sri Lanka. On 6 July 2010, Reuters reported:

"Sri Lanka's government is furious at Ban's appointment of the three-member panel on 22 June, saying it is a violation of its sovereignty and a hypocritical application of double standards by Western governments engaged in the war on terror...Sri Lanka is under pressure from the West, after rights watchdogs took advantage of the anniversary of the war's end to renew a push for an international probe into what they say are tens of thousands of civilian deaths."

This UN panel formed to conduct an inquiry on the war crimes had been refused visas to enter the country. "The Sri Lankan government promptly announced that it would not provide visas to the panel members to visit the country" (*Tamil News Network*, 12 July 2010).

Political tensions were further developing between the Canadian government and the Sri Lankan government on 13 August 2010 due to the arrival at Esquimalt, BC of the MV Sun Sea, a boat filled with 492 Tamil people seeking asylum in Canada. All made refugee claims citing violence in Sri Lanka.

The Sri Lankan government was suspicious of Canada, not only because of the large diaspora of Tamil people living in eastern Canada but also because Stephen Harper's conservative government was making war crime allegations against Sri Lanka.

With this news, it became more obvious why the government had blocked our visa. A Canadian ex-judge was not welcome in the country during this scrutiny for war crimes. I was a Canadian social worker wanting to work with the war affected. Naturally, the government did not want the stories of torture and violence to emerge.

It was possible that the work CUSO-VSO sought for us might be the actual barrier in obtaining visas. CUSO-VSO felt bad about the situation, calling it 'highly unusual'. But they were shrewd and believed that once we were inside the country, it might be easier to obtain clearance for the north.

They unlinked us from the Jaffna posting and worked on a new route of entry into Sri Lanka for us. We agreed to the new plan and CUSO started to look for a new partner organisation to work with in the south of Sri Lanka.

In the meantime, Bill and I began to study the reports on alleged war crimes. I soon realised that my personal trauma of my divorce was not the same as seeing your mother shot or your home burned or being forced to carry the decapitated head of your child during a forced march. I began to doubt my ability to help the Sri Lankan people.

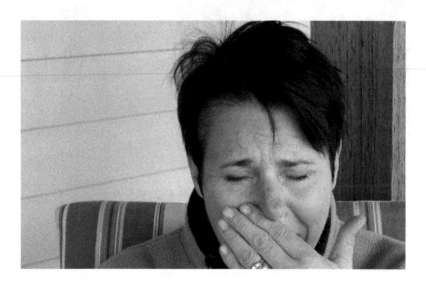

October 2010: Crying after the fourth cancellation of our Visa

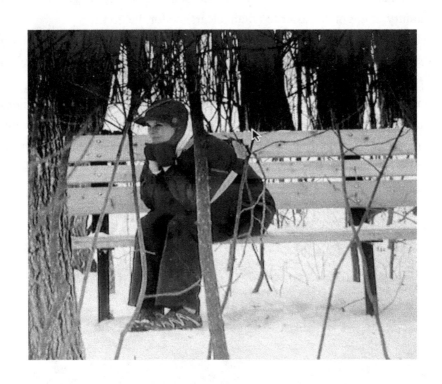

Winter 2010: The wait was getting to me

Chapter 7
Excitement Dampened by Grief

It is possible to experience both joy and loss at the same time. The soul's capacity to refract a myriad of human feelings at the same time is evidence of the divine.

On 21 November 2010, we received an email from CUSO that our visa clearance for the south of Sri Lanka had come through. We were booked to arrive in Colombo on 3 January 2011. The new partner organisation I was to work for was Nivahana Society of Kandy, Sri Lanka. *Kandy*, the name was synonymous with the exotic.

In celebration, we set up a tiny Christmas tree in the basement suite. These twinkling white lights symbolised our last Christmas in Canada for two years. We entertained friends we would not see again for two years and spent more time sorting, packing and repacking, deciding what and what not to take in terms of clothing, conveniences, food and books. We scooted about town trying to see all our family, as the days remaining in Canada were shrinking.

However, what took precedence over my time was visiting my dad. In June, my dad had had emergency surgery for an aortic aneurysm. While he pulled through the surgery, he was in bad shape. His breathing was laboured, shaking his entire body with each breath and his kidneys were shutting down.

The doctor counselled us that given dad's previous good health, it was worth a try to save him. Dad was intubated and hooked to a kidney dialysis machine. His breathing calmed and once the machine drained fluid from his body, he began to respond.

When he awoke, he seemed resurrected. He returned home and was stable for four months. However, his mobility was impaired and my mother was unable to care for him at home. He was moved into a rehabilitation facility and from there to the Hamlets, a supported living facility for further care. We all thought it was a temporary state.

One day, near Christmas, I decorated a tiny tree in his room at the Hamlets. Dad loved Christmas, and it was dismaying to see he didn't show much interest in the decorating. He seemed so apathetic and listless. That day, I hugged my dad goodbye and whispered into the folds of his stubbled neck, "Make sure you are still here when I get back."

He pushed me away and glared back into my eyes. "You make sure you get back," he growled, a tiny smile playing across his grey lips, his watery blue eyes twinkling. His feistiness relieved me.

It was clear. We both had directives for the next two years—him to stay healthy and alive and for me to get home to Canada in one piece. My relief proved short-lived.

In a few days, his feet turned black and he was re-hospitalised for ultrasound tests. His behaviour became more worrisome. Agitated, he began plucking at his blue hospital gown, his mumblings were incoherent and his eyes were casting about in a strange, paranoid manner. We thought his pain medication was the problem.

The ultrasound test results came in a few days later. There was severe loss of blood flow to the feet. Amputation of legs the suggested cure. I knew my father understood the difficulties of amputation as his own mother had lost her leg to gangrene, a complication of her diabetic condition.

The next day, heading to the hospital to visit Dad, I had my little five-year-old granddaughter, Lainee, with me. I noticed I still had a rosary in the ashtray of the car. I handed her the rosary. As she had had no religious training, I explained the rosary was a means to pray for assistance from the mother of Jesus. I told her to keep it and if she was ever frightened or worried about something, she could ask Jesus' mother to pray for her and she would feel better.

We rode the elevator to my dad's room on the medical ward of Royal Inland Hospital. He was in some sort of deep sleep. I peeked under the edge of the blankets and his blackened feet made me shudder. Lainee perched on a green vinyl chair at the end of his hospital bed and I crawled up onto the bed beside my dad.

I laid back against the rubbery pillow and put my arm around his barrel chest. He didn't move. I began to weep and whispered into his ear, "Dad, tell us what you want us to do." He did not flinch. He just breathed in his sleep.

"Dad," I implored, "Do you want us to fight for you or do you want us to let you go?"

I wept into the silence. Then, my precious little granddaughter walked around to the side of the bed and said, "Grandma, maybe Grandpa needs this." The rosary dangled from her small hand.

I smiled at her through my tears as I reached for the rosary. "I think you are right. That is what Grandpa needs."

Lainee crawled up onto the bed with me and I began the familiar and comforting litany of the rosary. The meditative quality of the repeated refrains, *Hail Mary, full of grace, The Lord is with you*, soothed me. When I was finished, I rested against my dad and in a ragged voice sang *Du, Du*, a German song he had sung to us as children.

His doctor assessed him that afternoon. "Your dad is in a coma, Wendy. He is now palliative. I will see about having him transferred to the palliative care home today." Seeing my stricken face, she added with compassion, "I am sorry, Wendy."

That night, my dad was moved to the Marjorie Snowden Palliative Care House. The family grapevine took over and within a couple of hours, our mother, seven of his eight children and some of the older grandchildren gathered around the single bed in the palliative care home. My father slept, his previously stubbled face now razored clean by the tender caring of a palliative nurse.

He was robed in a brown gown and looked like a holy friar in repose. Seeing my father like that reminded me again of his goodness and gentleness. Love gushed from me like tree sap from a sugar maple, draining me but somehow sweet too.

Later that evening, as the hour grew late, my mother crawled into the small hospital bed where my father lay breathing. Slowly, she lowered her small body down beside him as she had done for the past sixty years within the sanctity of their bedroom. Smoothing out stray wisps from dad's comb-over and placing her head on his pillow, she slowly stretched her arm up and over his chest.

She tucked her worn hand around the side of his rib cage, the thin wedding ring glinting in the muted shadows of the deepening night. Touched and fragile, we watched, witnesses to a wonderful marriage that was now about to end in a palliative care bed.

Me, my brothers and sisters and some of the older grandchildren surrounded his bed, some on chairs, some sitting on the floor, some with hoodies pulled up over their heads, others drawing inward. Each of us huddled down into our own grief. We wept and waited. My mother led a rosary.

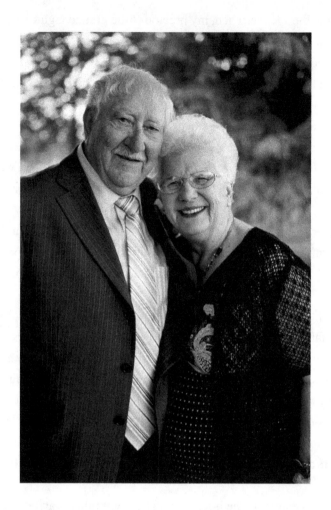

My Mother and Father: On the day of their 60th wedding anniversary, just six months before the death of my father

We supervised his breathing. Long lapses existed between breaths, and we were both relieved and dismayed each time he gasped for another breath of life.

Nearing morning and fearing the time was near, my eldest brother, Glenn, the only one of us not in the room, was teleconferenced in from Kingston, Ontario, 4600 kilometres away, to say his own goodbye. Glenn choked out over the speakerphone, "Dad, you were a good father. You led an exemplary and honourable life. I love you."

With that simple and touching affirmation, Dad drew his last breath. It was first light on 20 December 2010. It was ironic that we prayed for him to not linger but could never prepare ourselves for the blow of that last breath. The sob that erupted from one of my most silent brothers was our collective cry of grief.

The fragility of life and the permanence of death was devastating. Grief left me shaken and fragile, but also, unfettered to depart. Ten days later, on 3 January 2011, Bill and I boarded a plane, leaving Canada for Sri Lanka.

Part Two
Warm-Up in Freezing Hill Country

Chapter 8
Arriving in Colombo

When a life event takes place, we sometimes ponder; was it pre-ordained,
accidental or planned? Often it is a magical brew of all three.

On 4 January 2011, we landed at Bandaranayke Airport in Colombo. The flight was a gruelling twenty-two hours in the air. Although I had followed a colleague's advice and swallowed Melatonin, as night approached mid-air, I didn't sleep.

In contrast, Bill slept like a baby. I found his gaping open mouth a bit much to look at for such a long time. The hours of inactivity on a cramped plane filled my ankles like camel humps, my hands resembling pork sausage links. I climbed off the plane punch-drunk and disoriented. Heat and humidity slapped me in the face.

Wavering through the busy airport, we focused on signs written in English, found amongst the squiggled curlicues of the Sinhala alphabet and the stronger, thicker lines of the Tamil alphabet. We located the baggage carousel where our bulging Asolo packs cycled out of the loading dock onto the airport's baggage claim conveyor.

Stuffed inside our bags were our possessions for two years and they were already melding together in the heat. Sweat trickled down our backs, soaking the waistband of our shorts as we lugged our packs towards the concourse, dodging harried women in colourful saris who tugged along children, bundles, cartons and suitcases.

Men with bushy eyebrows furrowing with anxiety rushed to meet their scheduled flights. Some of the men wore sarongs and others wore trousers. Some carried children, but others resembled beasts of burden as they hoisted beaten travelling trunks onto their backs before hurrying along.

Bill and I lumbered towards the exit under the weight of the packs. Feeling anxious, we gawked around, hoping to see the VSO people that were supposed to be there to pick us up.

Outside the airport, throngs of tour guides, relatives of travellers, trishaw and taxi drivers waved signs and were calling aloud: Lanka Tours, Sun Fun Vacations, Kandy Tourist Services, Themala and Malli Weerasinghe and Perera Family. We spotted a sign that read:

Bill and Wendy
VSO

A tall, slender man and a woman dressed in red were smiling and waving the sign. Shyly, we approached. "Aayuboovan," said the woman, bowing at the waist. She introduced herself as Manchula, the VSO officer we had been communicating with regarding our visa clearance.

Manchula's luxurious black hair waved down to her shoulder blades. Rhinestones studded her red shalwar. She was tiny and beautiful, not what I had expected of a legal compliance officer. She shook our hands as did Upali, the VSO transport officer.

Upali was fit and handsome in an immaculate white shirt. His slacks, creased like a knife blade, would impress any naval officer. He stashed our monstrous backpacks into the spacious Land Rover, and we ducked inside the cool, air-conditioned vehicle.

As we headed out into the traffic, we noticed that oxen and carts, cows, trishaws, motorcycles, mopeds, tractors, ice cream carts, cycle bikes and pedestrians shared the road. Colourfully dressed people picked their way along uprooted sidewalks. Trishaws beeped at every turn, dancing in and out of traffic. Larger vehicles ploughed through the traffic, blaring horns and creating an opening like the Red Sea.

Tambilli (apricot-coloured) coconuts dangled from storefront beams or squatted in the sun on the pavement outside of the small shops along our route. Palm trees lined the streets and stood swaying in the breeze off the Indian Ocean. We swooned as the exotic smell of rot, salt and cinnamon assailed us. We sat close, holding hands in the back seat, silently reassuring one another.

Ten minutes into our drive, Manchula turned to us and asked if we needed water. We both nodded. The heat was wringing water from our bodies, soaking our clothing. Upali pulled up to a small store.

Inside was an untidy jumble of unknown products, with labels we couldn't read, bottles and containers we didn't recognise and an order to shelving that defied logic. We could have selected poison for all we knew.

Manchula led us to a cooler near the back of the store and we selected water bottles. As Manchula paid for our drinks, we gazed around the store. Elbowing me, Bill nodded his head towards a sign above a large doorframe that led to another dinghy but smaller room within the store. The room was shelved with recognisable bottles of alcohol: Bombay gin, Canadian whiskey, Australian wine, Russian vodka and other liquor.

The crooked sign Bill had indicated dangled from a piece of binder twine hooked over a nail partially driven into the doorframe. The proprietor of the store had written in English with a black felt pen on a yellowed piece of cardboard.

We do not sell arrack to ladies.

Bill snickered. We both assumed arrack was alcohol. He was going to have to be my bootlegger. Why were we not forewarned about this important detail? I felt some concern.

Back in the car, we passed through Borella Junction, a roundabout with dizzying spurs. A thundering din from heavy vehicular and pedestrian traffic arose as Upali steered the vehicle into Cotta Road, then made a right-hand turn down a narrow lane. A large wrought iron gate loomed at the end of the lane, and as the Land Rover approached, a security guard emerged from a tiny booth on the other side and slid open the gate for us to pass.

Inside the gate, an elegant ranch-style house stood amidst wide-bladed green grass and a riot of brilliant flowering shrubs. Palm and coconut trees hung heavy with their fruit. As we creaked out of the Land Rover, fat insects hummed, stupefied by the heat. An old rusty bike leaned against the porch of the house.

Manchula escorted us inside the house that had been converted into the VSO headquarters for Sri Lanka. The wide vestibule was blessedly cool. Lining the walls sat a lending library stacked with classics, fiction, non-fiction, autobiographies, travel books and DVDs such as *Grey's Anatomy*, *The West Wing* and *Downton Abbey*.

At the far end of the vestibule, a receptionist named Angela was seated at a desk. She greeted us and advised us to contact her if we needed anything during our stay. We were also introduced to Anusha, the VSO volunteer youth advisor, and Ruvanthi, the VSO program office director. We were led into the large dining area. Lal, the tiny, sinewy VSO cook greeted us with a broad, toothless smile.

"Come, come," he bowed and waved his small brown hand up and down as if patting a child on the head. He beckoned us to sit at the large dining table covered in clear plastic. Chatting to us in Sinhala, he boiled up the electric kettle and thrust steaming mugs of milk tea at us. Even though we had no idea what he was saying, we smiled awkwardly.

We sipped the caramel-coloured mixture of orange pekoe tea, powdered cream and tablespoons of sugar. Despite the heat, the hot sweet milky tea was exactly what we needed—it boosted our blood sugars.

"Thank you, sir," Bill said a bit too bright, shifting his eyes to mine, begging me to say something too. I sat mute. It was so awkward not to be able to communicate. Soon, Upali returned to drive us to our accommodation.

"Your guesthouse is called Chelsea Gardens. It will be your temporary residence while you go through your three week in-country induction training," he said.

Colombo is numbered into fifteen postal districts. Chelsea Gardens sat in the heart of Colombo 3, also known as Kollupitiya, which is one of the main commercial areas of the city and the home of the exotic Cinnamon Gardens and their vast mansions from the colonial era. The guesthouse was owned and operated by Mrs Padmini Nanayakkara, a tall, elegant older Sri Lankan woman.

Padmini spoke the Queen's English. She ushered us into her home furnished in teak, with fine china and numerous framed family photos alongside paintings of countryside.

By this time, we had been up for more than thirty hours and it had been some time since our last meal. Padmini's housekeeper scrambled eggs and served them in the tiny courtyard garden. Padmini poured strong tea from a china teapot and with fine silver tongs she plopped sweet amber nuggets of cane sugar called jaggery into our teacups. We ate to nourish ourselves, but we longed to lie down and sleep.

Padmini ushered us upstairs into a spacious and well-lit room in her guesthouse. "This is the matrimonial room," she explained, gesturing to the large double bed in the middle of the room. Draping the bed was a bright, woven coverlet. A tiny ensuite bathroom with a shower sat off the bedroom.

Handing us the keys, Padmini said goodnight, although it was ten o'clock in the morning, and rustled away. Dead tired, we undressed, leaving our soggy clothes in a heap on the floor.

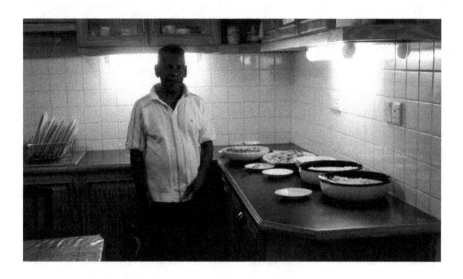

Lal with his wonderful food creations in the VSO office in Colombo

Anticipating the luxury of sleep, we pulled back the coverlet. Bill and I exchanged grimaces. Two single beds had been shoved together, each made with individual top and bottom sheets. The striped cotton bedspread placed over both the beds created the illusion of a double bed.

Our custom of sleeping in each other's arms seemed about to change. We climbed into our own narrow bed and hugged over the crevice.

Again, Bill slept well. My nervous system jerked me awake again and again just as I was about to fall asleep. I hadn't slept well since Dad's death. My vulnerability at the loss evidenced in my disrupted sleeps. Yet, I did not miss him.

When he was alive, it was as if he was over there, in his house, somewhere. Now that he had died, I had embodied him somehow and he now lived inside or had become a part of me, never having left. His spirit was with me, supporting my journey.

Around nine o'clock that evening, we arose, showered and ventured into the dark streets near the guesthouse. Timid to wander too far in such an unfamiliar place, we circled about, trying to locate a restaurant open late on a Sunday night. We spied a restaurant. The menu was strange to us, and we ended up ordering egg hoppers.

They resembled a very thin white rice crepe pressed into the shape of a cereal bowl and infused with a fried egg. They were delicious! After dinner, we retraced our steps home grateful for the light from the infrequent streetlamps. Cockroaches scurried about our feet in the dark as we did our own scurrying back to the safety of our guesthouse.

We entered the gloom of the garage under the apartment. It was empty, other than a couple of cockroaches and a large chunk of cardboard strewn in the far corner. Peering into the dark, we realised that upon the cardboard was a ragged, greying blanket covering a tiny, elderly man curled up and asleep. We were stunned. We were to learn that he was the security guard for the building and saw him every night we stayed there.

As the morning sun streamed through the window, Stanley, another driver, fetched us from Chelsea Gardens to start our in-country orientation at the VSO office. Following staff introductions, we scribbled out paperwork necessary for the Canadian and British Embassy, received security clearance ID badges, opened a local bank account, and had our university degrees photocopied.

We had been asked to bring our original degrees from Canada as well as our marriage certificate, an important document in Sri Lanka. These precious documents were stored in the VSO safe.

Other volunteers in our training group included Dr Kamal Kainth, a psychologist from London. Kamal was assigned to work for the same organisation I had been assigned, The Nivahana Society of Kandy. We also met Venus Samson, a woman from the Philippines, skilled in social service work. Anne Murray, a business consultant from Scotland arrived a few days later.

Our training included orientation on the political situation, the governmental structure and gender issues, along with intensive language training in the Sinhala language. Afterwards, we set out to make some necessary purchases: a Nokia cell phone, an adapter to run our computers and a blow dryer that worked on 220 voltage. My inner thighs were chafing from the heat and so I purchased a pair of shorts for under my skirts. We were roasting alive.

The next day, we began language lessons with Ianthi, our Sinhala teacher. She was an outgoing middle-aged woman, who assisted us with the alphabet and simple phrases to assist us with greetings, discussions about family and shopping in the market. One day, Ianthi ordered trishaws for us all to enter the chaos of Pettah Market to learn the names of dangling fruits, stacked tomatoes, chickens with flies and fish on ice.

Tea and cloth vendors enticed us into their stores while exotic birds shrieked at us as we passed. In awe, we watched Ianthi purchasing spice from plastic bins piled to the brim with orange cumin, yellow curry and red pepper. She selected potatoes and eggplant and zucchini, bargaining in Sinhala with all her might with the vendors.

Our visit to the market was not incident-free. In the jumble and commotion of Pettah, a man in the bustling tea market groped Bill. Bill confessed he felt a bit victimised by the experience. From our VSO gender training, we both realised this was the everyday experience of many Sri Lankan women.

Lal did the cooking lessons and lunch preparation. With the ingredients Ianthi had selected in the market, Lal worked in his tiny kitchen, teaching us his methods for cooking Sri Lankan food. When he was done, a vat of white rice sat alongside four different curries on the counter, buffet style. A spicy relish called sambal was offered for flavour. Laying out our food, Lal sounded a gong and we lined up along with the VSO staff to eat.

We ate the delicious food with our forks. I watched Anusha, one of the VSO staff eat her lunch. Picking up some sambal from her plate, she dropped it down on some rice. She selected a chicken curry and dropped it on the sambal. Next, she placed a brinjal curry on top of the chicken curry.

Fascinated, I stared as her right hand started to mash the food together between thumb and fingers. Press, mash and massage. Press, mash, massage. Mixing food with the right hand is an important part of eating in the Sri Lankan culture, but we didn't know that then.

Anusha conversed in Sinhala to her colleague all the while, who was also pressing, mashing and massaging her food. Then, once the food reached a gluey texture, she formed a loose ball, held it in her fingers and then, out jumped her thumb, pushing the food ball into her mouth. She waved her littered hand about as she spoke. I tried not to focus on the mucky rice sticking like maggots on her hand. A need to gag arose.

By the end of the training, we began to feel like we were the odd ones, eating with forks. So, I sunk my hands into the yellow curry and rice and began mashing. I loved it! I never again ate Sri Lankan food any other way. Bill tried to be game about it, but he remained squeamish and over time developed a distinct dislike for Sri Lankan curry. He just couldn't stomach fish curry for breakfast and curry again for lunch and dinner.

Our training narrowed focus, and Ruvanthi, the in-country manager, provided more information about our organisation. The Nivahana Society of Kandy partnered with VSO and the Sri Lankan Ministry of Health to develop primary, secondary and tertiary mental health services. As she began referring to a hospital, I kept hearing the words "nuwa elya."

"What is that?" I asked, my confusion evident. Bill cocked his head as well.

"What is what?" Ruvanthi asked.

"Those two words you keep saying," I pressed.

"What two words?" Ruvanthi raised her eyebrows and peered over her eyeglasses at me.

"Nuwa elya," I stumbled.

"Nuwara Eliya? Why, that is where you are going!" Ruvanthi looked back at us, puzzled.

"No," I stated, shaking my head. "We are going to Kandy. You know, the Nivahana Society of Kandy."

Ruvanthi chuckled. "I thought you knew that. Nivahana Society is not in Kandy but in Nuwara Eliya. You are going there."

We gaped at her. We had researched Kandy. We hadn't researched Nuwara Eliya. We had never even heard of the place. We couldn't even pronounce it.

"It is very cold there," snickered Upali, who had just overheard the conversation as he entered the room.

"We are from Canada. It is not cold for us," we joshed to be good sports, but concern approached. We felt like unprepared Boy Scouts heading into a storm.

Not realising how much she had unnerved us, Ruvanthi carried on. She explained that the psychiatric unit at Nuwara Eliya General Hospital was only two years old, as was the outpatient psychiatric clinic attached to the hospital. My role was to support and train the staff in reducing stigma of mental health, train staff on the bio-psychosocial model of mental health practice and improve the conditions of the patients and the mentally ill in the community.

Near the end of our induction, Ruvanthi pulled Bill aside. "Bill, I have not forgotten about you, but to date, have been unable to locate a position for you. I don't know why it is so difficult, but I promise I will find you a job."

Bill was disappointed. He had already shared with me that he couldn't help feeling a little less valued than the other volunteers. "I'm a bit of a tag-along," he confessed. He assured Ruvanthi he was willing to wait for a position but made it clear that any position he held would need to be in the same town as mine.

In the remaining days of our training, our language lessons continued. Armed with the alphabet and some basic words and phrases such as days of the week, numbers and shopping terms, we practiced with each other and in the nearby shops and restaurants. After hours, we explored the capital city of Colombo, in the country most of us would call home for the next two years.

Chapter 9
Nesting in Our New Mountain Home

A home is not a house. It is a feeling, familiar and constant. It is a smell, a safety imbued into the very walls.

After three weeks of training and language lessons, it was time to begin our work. Upali picked us up and helped heave our heavy bags down the stairs from Padmini's guesthouse. We slogged through the traffic past the populated districts of Colombo until the buildings thinned.

We moved past low wooden and corrugated metal shanties and colourful vegetable stands alongside the narrow road, ushered along by the rich green foliage that swayed as we passed on our way into the interior of Sri Lanka. We stopped for the night in Kandy.

Upali secured a guesthouse overlooking the tiny lake around which hilly Kandy is built. The guesthouse was run by a genteel Sinhalese woman, Mrs Jayasinghe, who provided us a delicious meal of rice and curries. Before retiring, she instructed us to keep the windows closed.

As the orange sun glowed through the morning mist, thundering on the metal roof of the guesthouse awakened us. Still in bed, we assumed this noise was a thunder and lightning storm.

"Wendy, look," Bill whispered, pointing to the window at the end of our bed. A small black hand gripped a bar on our window. I was in shock. We looked out the other windows, all of which had wrought iron bars across them.

Monkeys flew past, capering along the railings and screeching at each other along the rooftops, rattling the corrugated roofing that thundered into our room. The monkeys seemed to be demanding a take-over of the house. It felt a bit frightening and foreign. *Are these creatures going to be near our new home?* we asked ourselves as we fled downstairs to breakfast.

After a refreshing breakfast of papaya, buffalo curd and fried eggs, we headed deeper into Hill Country. As we trundled past Kandy, we began a steep ascent along the narrow highway into the mountains. Gentle banana palms moved their fronds back and forth, and tiny roadside shanties featured signs offering bhat (rice) takeaways. As we climbed on, the lush, warm forests of Kandy started to disappear and well-trimmed tea plantations and vegetable stands took their place over the hilly landscape.

Cool mist fingered the forests and plantations. It was both eerie and haunting. Misty waterfalls splashed down ravines between the mountains like something ethereal. Deep, cold pools formed at the bottom of the falls and were filled with people bathing or washing vegetables for market.

We shivered as the temperature continued to drop and snuggled deeper into the flimsy tropical clothing we'd donned the previous day in steamy hot Colombo. Colombo already felt like a long way away. Fear and uncertainty settled upon us we zigzagged high into the mountain.

Just a few kilometres outside of Nuwara Eliya, the fan belt snapped on the Land Rover. Upali hopped out, flipped open the hood and inspected the motor. He wiggled a few wires and hoses, then in disgust, flagged down a passing trishaw, arranged payment and had the trishaw driver take us into town.

As we drove into town, we noticed men with heads wrapped in long woollen scarves tied like turbans, while women wore wool scarves draped over their heads and tied under the chin or one end thrown up over the shoulder. Serviceable grey and brown woollen sweaters and fleece hoodies were donned over women's saris while men wore the hoodies and sweaters with their plaid sarongs. The locals seemed overdressed for the weather which we understood only later.

We checked into our guesthouse, the Alpine Lodge. Upali arranged for repair of the vehicle and told us that in the morning we should begin the search for a place to live.

Fear struck us. Our Sinhala was horrible. In language school, we had learned the names of useful things like eloolu (vegetables) and palatura (fruits), but had failed to learn necessary terminology for renting like: "Do the stove, fridge, furnishings, beds and such come with the house? Does it have air conditioning? Are utilities included?"

Beside our linguistic shortcomings, we had limited money, and we didn't know the region. We begged Upali to help us before he returned to Colombo. Seeing our desperation, he took pity on us and engaged himself as our negotiator, suite finder and translator.

The next morning over breakfast Upali explained, "Sri Lankan people are leery of renting. They hold a belief that renters can acquire squatter's rights. The land they own is often referred to as ancient land as it was passed along over many generations."

He shoved a ball of mashed curry into his mouth, swallowing it down with a sip of milk tea. He continued, "They do not want to risk losing this ancient land. Therefore, there is very little property to rent." Bill and I looked at each other. We had been homeless long enough.

"However," Upali brightened, "they do like to rent to foreigners, as they assume foreigners will not stay long enough to acquire any squatter rights."

After breakfast, Upali wasted no time. He mentioned our dilemma to the deskman at the hotel. The deskman called his friend, who knew a friend who had a house. We looked at a total of ten places that morning.

I suspect many of the places had sat vacant for several years. Bill and I are not Molly Maids or obsessive about cleanliness, but grimy walls, thick dust and dark, mud-caked windows did not feel welcoming.

Most of the landlords we met that day assumed that we, as foreigners, had deep pockets, and led us to palatial homes we would have loved to rent. But the housing stipend provided by VSO limited luxury housing. Our rent ceiling was 30,000 Rs (rupees) for a furnished place and 25,000 Rs for a non-furnished place. This secured modest housing.

Most landlords, nonplussed by our declination of their property extended other useful services. I have a car rental place. My sister does laundry. My cousin can do some cooking. If you need anything, just come by. It was a gracious way to conduct business.

Upali led us to a little semi-furnished guest cottage on a property belonging to Sudu Malli and Deelu Perera. Sudu Malli's impish smile charmed me instantly, while Deelu, in advanced pregnancy, stood strong, chattering to us in Sinhala, oblivious to the fact that we didn't understand a word. Their girls, Tharushi and Malisha, who attended the Maghastota English School down the back lane, beamed while translating our conversation to their parents.

We had viewed one other property that was much closer to the hospital and the city centre, but Upali advised us, "In my opinion, the warmth and welcome of Sudu Malli's family made the extra ten minutes of commute to work worth your while." He was right.

Over milk tea in their spacious home situated on the hill behind our cottage, we shook hands on the rent price that was within the VSO budget. With this business transaction completed, Upali assisted us in unloading our bags from the Land Rover, along with some household furnishings he had extracted from the Colombo VSO garage, and waving, headed down into the mist.

We moved in. I shoved furniture into corners to create comfortable spaces, hung our wrinkled clothing in the tiny wooden closet and stacked pots and pans in our musky smelling kitchen. Bill sang off-key and shouted at the top of his lungs as he figured out how to light the pilot on the gas stove in the kitchen.

He strung a clothesline across the small yard and created a grocery list of necessary staples and sundries. We were looking forward to some calm and a sense of a home to prepare us for the next step of the real work in Sri Lanka.

We started to explore the town and its surroundings. Nuwara Eliya is a small town that nestles deep down in what is known as the Hill Country in the Central Province of Sri Lanka. Its name means 'City of the Plains' or 'City of Light'. It is situated at 6,128 feet (1,868 metres) above sea level, and three of the tallest mountains in Sri Lanka (Mount Pidurutalagal, Great Western and Haggala) soar around it.

These peaks house the rain forests of Sri Lanka and are often cloaked in a variegated, swirling grey mist. Standing on top of one of these mountains, on a rare day when the sun penetrates the mist, Lake Gregory can be spotted in a small mossy basin at the base of the mountains.

Rolling hills of tea plantations surround the lake. Lush tea plants were spaced and neatly trimmed into tabletops resembling lime green coffee tables. On the rare day of sun, each tea bush is draped with shirts and sarongs, underpants and blouses laid out to dry.

Nuwara Eliya's tea is an important Sri Lankan agricultural commodity used both domestically and for export. Nuwara Eliya also survives on the proceeds from a golf course, the Hakgala Botanical Gardens and horse racing on a lumpy, horse-tripping-hazard racetrack.

It was here that Bill and I settled into our tiny two-bedroom home. A newer building, it was fresh and clean. The living and dining area were one long room, and off this was a small kitchen. The kitchen's big bright windows faced a lush green lawn confined by a concrete garden wall.

Above the wall sat a lime green hill covered in tea plants and dotted with corrugated sheet metal shanty homes. In the two bathrooms, tiny hot water tanks were affixed to the walls high above the shower spout. The walls above were concrete and whitewashed.

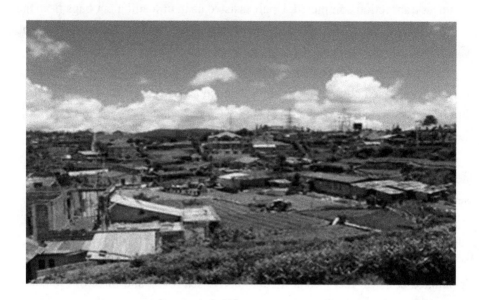

Our neighbourhood in Nuwara Eliya. Our cottage was below the large home at the back/middle of photo

Our bed thrilled us. It was a double bed with a double mattress, a true 'matrimonial' bed. It was brand new, still covered in plastic with the mattress edges encased in heavy chunks of cardboard. That first evening, before pulling on our new bed sheets, Bill and I sat on the bed, scratching our heads.

"Should we remove the plastic?" Bill wondered.

"Do you think it was meant to be left on?" I queried.

We knew we didn't want to hear the crinkling and rustling of plastic every time we moved at night. So, we hedged our bets. Bill fetched a kitchen knife and slit the plastic covering on one full length of the mattress and both ends. Then, stripping the plastic back off the mattress, we stuffed it between the bed's sideboard and the mattress for safekeeping. We crawled in under the covers, snuggled, feeling safe and settled.

Two weeks after we moved in, our landlady, Deelu, invited us up for tea and biscuits. At one point during the evening, her new-born son was howling for a needed diaper change. Deelu gestured for me to follow her into her bedroom while she changed the baby.

Uncomfortable in this private place, I lowered my bottom onto the bed. It was greeted with a loud rustle. In horror, I shifted slightly. Crinkle. Crinkle. After the tea party, Bill and I hopped on our scooter and sped to the local hardware store for duct tape.

Through VSO, we had learned the broad strokes of the culture but had much to learn about the fine brush strokes within the domestic realm of a culture.

Chapter 10
Starting My Volunteer Work

In this strange land of unusual weather and dilapidated buildings, there was one cheer, a smiling face.

At six o'clock in the morning the alarm rattled me from my woollen cocoon of blankets. Groaning and steeling myself against the cold, I threw my legs over the side of the bed and put my feet, encased in wool socks, down on the cold tile. Pulling my toque down over my ears, I shuffled into the kitchen to heat the kettle and then shuffled back into the tiny bathroom to start my miserable shower.

In the kitchen, Bill stirred thick porridge laced with coconut milk and cardamom. He boiled coffee while I showered. I missed the leisure of retirement. By the time we arrived in Nuwara Eliya, I had not worked for a year. We had galivanted the entire year of 2010.

After breakfast, I donned my rain pants and rain poncho, wiped the puddle from the black vinyl seat of my scooter, straddled it and turned the bike into the driving rain. I headed down muddy Vijithapura by-road that dipped onto the main highway into town.

With grey mist lifting off Lake Gregory on my right, I slowed my bike for sleek brown racehorses fornicating on the main road near the racetrack that stood on the outskirt of town. Then, turning right, I headed towards Hawa Eliya, a suburb of Nuwara Eliya, where the hospital was located. I was nervous. It was my first day of work.

I had been instructed to wait at the main gate of the hospital. I steered my bike into the mucky pull-off, and there I parked my splattered blue scooter in the mud. Still astraddle, coated in plastic rain gear, I peered about as I waited.

Inside the main gate I could see low, shabby buildings with peeling yellowed paint. Scruffy plants grew helter-skelter around the property. Dreary vending stands stood along one of the muddy streets that separated the buildings.

Umbrellas bobbed along the grounds of the hospital streets; people were packing howling children in their arms or attempting to push rickety wheelchairs filled with listless elderly through the mud. I felt subdued and disoriented by the sheer poverty and the lack of a clinical presence that I was used to in a hospital.

A tiny nurse approached me. Her step was dainty as she picked her way along the rutted road, avoiding the deeper puddles. Her hair was in a large, braided bun that supported an even larger white nursing cap. She wore a white nursing uniform with a striped white and navy apron and shoes, polished to a dull white.

White calf length socks covered her twiggy legs. Her large brown eyes peered out from under the metallic points of her huge navy umbrella.

"Dr Windy?" My lips twitched into a smile.

"Yes, hello. Are you Chamali?"

"Yes," Chamali giggled, her enormous smile capturing me. I slid off my scooter, my foot sinking into the mud. "Come, follow me." She crooked her finger towards the buildings to the far right of the gate.

A sliver of white gold on her ring finger indicated that she was married. I was grateful that she spoke English. I was already feeling overwhelmed by the decrepit looking hospital site.

Chamali conducted a vivacious orientation as we sloshed along. "The hospital is a set of old buildings that, in the past, was the site of the Lion Beer Brewing Company. Many years ago, the brewing company moved their operation to Colombo, leaving the buildings vacant. They were then taken over by the government for the General Hospital."

Pointing with her tiny forefinger, she continued, "That is the main hospital, where Admitting, Emergency and the Surgical Theatre are situated. The Medical wards and Maternity wards are there as well."

As we walked along the muddy street, several sick and mangy dogs trudged past us, heading somewhere. Chamali seemed not to notice. "These shops," she pointed to a row of low wooden stalls such as you might see at a fall fair that have been constructed to sell seasonal pies, "are where you can buy lunch packets and gifts for patients."

As we rounded the corner, she pointed out the Diabetic Clinic and the Medical Clinic. The Medical Clinic had several rows of rough wooden benches outside the small wooden building. The benches were filling with people, striking in their thinness and bundled with woollen turbans or scarves tied under angular chins.

Nobody smiled or seemed to speak. They sat in the drizzle, glum but determined. It all seemed so unfamiliar. I pulled at my coat, wrapping it closer.

"Here we are," Chamali said. A long, whitewashed building stood to the left of where we were standing. It was barrack-like with barred windows equidistance from the other. "That is the Psychiatric ward," she explained. Damp leaves and bits of paper blown by the cold wind were swirling into a corner where a broken concrete wall butted up to the hospital building.

"That, over there," she gestured with her tiny hand, "is the Mental Health Outpatient Clinic." A small, shabby concrete building stood across the alley from the main psychiatric ward. "Dr Ajith Navaratne is our chief psychiatrist," she explained, dark eyes glistening. "He has asked me to greet you and show you to his office."

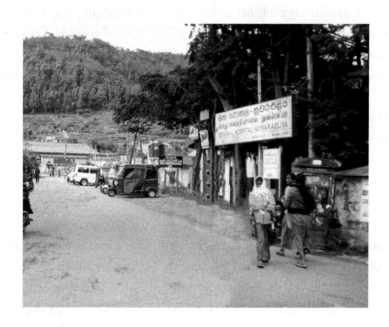

General Hospital in Nuwara Eliya

She leaned her small body against a large metal door that gave way with ease. In our muddy shoes, we stepped across the threshold into the dark concrete vestibule of the psychiatric ward. Chamali pointed to a small office. "This is Dr Ajith's office," she said. "You can wait here. I will bring you some tea."

I shifted in the white plastic chair I had been offered. I glanced about at the starkness of the office, trying not to compare or judge. A computer tower was perched upon the enormous grey metal desk. The window was covered in a limp, faded green curtain. An ancient dot matrix printer sat below the window on grey metal shelving.

Dr Ajith bustled into the office. "Dr Windy, welcome. Not the best weather to greet you, is it?" I wrinkled my nose in agreement. I suddenly felt at ease. He seemed affable and intelligent. Unruly curls sat atop his head, and his eyes sparkled with mirth.

Chamali re-entered the office, bearing a silver tray with tiny teacups brimming with tea and laced with sugar and milk. I began to thaw out as the warm amber liquid penetrated the chill in my body. As we sipped, they inquired about my education and experience.

I reciprocated with my own inquiries about the hospital and the expectations they had for me. As we finished our tea, Dr Ajith suggested a tour of the ward, followed by their scheduled patient rounds.

We moved through a locked door into a large, open hospital room. It looked like CNN television clips of hospitals in the developing world. The windows were all barred. The whole ward was dark and dank, and the muddy green paint coating the rough concrete did little to brighten it.

Patients dressed in street clothes huddled into themselves on old metal frame beds cushioned by two-inch foam pads and covered in striped fabric. There were no drapes between the beds to even suggest a sense of privacy. The ward was barren and devoid of chairs, tables, pictures, or curtains.

Not everyone had a blanket even though the ward was freezing. Patients without blankets sat on their beds hunched or lay in a foetal position on the bed, arms wrapping their legs for warmth. Chamali explained that blankets and food were not provided by the hospital, but by the patient's family.

In the hospital I worked for in Canada, patients were either in rooms with four beds or had semi-private rooms. Hospital beds draped with linens and blankets sat next to reading lamps and bedside tables. Rooms were bright and clean, and patients were free to wander about the ward, to go outside into a green-space courtyard and to help themselves to snacks in the fridge. The coffee pot was on all day long. Books, puzzles, drawing materials, television and programs like occupational therapy, psychoeducation, group and individual therapy were available every day. It was a stark contrast.

My stomach felt queasy, and I took furtive glances about as Dr Ajith described the history of the hospital. "This psychiatric ward opened just two years ago. It is a twenty-bed adult ward with no seclusion or special care unit. Thus, psychotic or violent patients are not admitted but sent to Kandy hospital."

"The ward is divided into the men's ward and the women's ward. Both are locked, and no intermingling exists between the men and women. Children admitted to the psychiatric ward are placed on the female side of the ward, but we prefer sending them to the hospital in Kandy," he explained as we moved throughout the ward.

A handsome man in his forties sat slumped on the edge of his bed and barely lifted his head to respond to the doctor. He stared, then blinked, a weak acknowledgement. Dr Ajith explained, "He was catatonic when brought to hospital. However, he is slowly improving."

An elderly man paced about the ward like a caged tiger, uttering quiet threats, his eyes darting and suspicious. Possibly dementia, I noted to myself. Another man, unshaven and dishevelled, believed he was being persecuted by the devil. His family, no longer able to manage him, had brought him to the hospital. He sat mumbling to himself, responding to inner stimuli.

In the female ward, a woman in a blue sari sat cross-legged on her bed. Her speech was pressured and rapid and her smile provocative as the doctor explained to me that she had a bipolar mood disorder and was in a manic phase. Another large woman, dressed in a dishevelled sari, sang under her breath but smiled, flashing crooked teeth marred with severe dental caries.

We exited the ward, locking the door behind us. Female nurses in white caps and uniforms and male nurses in white lab coats sat in a small, barred office and observed patients through the iron bars. They hand-documented their clinical notes in large file ledgers, one for each patient. I observed they did not speak to patients.

As we walked back to his office, Dr Ajith explained more about mental illness in Sri Lanka. Due to the stigma and lack of education about the nature of mental illness, few referrals are made to psychiatry early in the progression of the illness. Families have strong concerns about bringing a patient for treatment as it affects eligibility for marriage.

If a woman is mentally ill, she becomes a 'risky' choice and her chances of securing a good husband are diminished while the dowry demands are increased, further burdening the family. Males with mental illness may not be offered a wife if the woman's family have concerns for their daughter. As a result, often, by the time a person presents for treatment, their symptoms are very severe and require hospitalisation.

Dr Ajith invited me to attend his outpatient clinic. While beckoning the male orderly to start allowing patients in one by one, Dr Ajith explained that at that time, Sri Lanka had the highest suicide rate in the world. In 2012, almost four thousand people took their own lives.

He told me that poverty, joblessness, debt and social problems all contributed to the high rates of suicide. In addition, a cultural component permeates. Sri Lanka, as other Asian countries, has a face-saving society. Women ostracised by their family and community after being 'defiled' through rape, therefore, not eligible for marriage, often turn to suicide to save face for themselves and their family.

Women who have no dowry commit suicide to avoid remaining a burden to the family members as spinsters. Women believe they have no value if not married. They commit suicide by swallowing pesticides, hanging and self-immolation.

Employment is very difficult to secure in Sri Lanka. Men, still the primary provider of the family, often feel shame and turn to alcohol abuse or suicide when they cannot meet the economic needs of the family. I listened, adopting an attitude of curiosity and assessment. I asked more questions and took more notes.

At home at night, snuggling up to Bill, I reviewed my notes. Functional nursing care seemed to include medication and charting. Nurses appeared well-trained in general nursing practice but had no training in psychiatry, psychiatric patient care, family work, or how to communicate with mentally ill patients.

It distressed me that the nurses remained in the nursing station for the most part and entered the ward only when necessary. Patients were sitting upon their beds with no stimulation other than the family member who often sat with them. Many just lay on their beds or stared out the window. There was no programming, crafts, television, snacks, books, or paper.

I was an experienced mental health professional. I had seen acute mental illness, psychosis, major depression and addiction every day at the hospital. Mental illness and severity of illness did not shock me. Neither did the myriad of manifestations of human mental illness bother me.

What *did* shock me was that many of the patients here looked to me like they no longer possessed a soul. They seemed devoid of hope. I had not seen that look of despair before. It haunted me. My mind began percolating ideas for training.

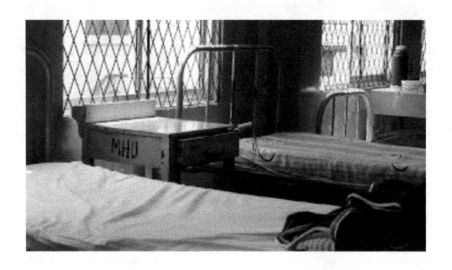

Psychiatric Ward, General Hospital Nuwara Eliya

The hospital in Nuwara Eliya had never had a VSO volunteer before. They did not know what a volunteer could offer or how they could help. My job description was open, and it was up to me to figure out how I might make a difference.

For the next two months, I assessed the organisation. I followed Ajith, Chamali and the three other physicians around the ward. In the vestibule, I attended assessments where patients were lined up outside the psychiatrist's office, the doors and windows open to the lobby inside where privacy could be breached by staff or patients.

The doctor heard the story from the patient or a family member, made a diagnosis and determined as to whether to admit the patient to hospital or treat them as an outpatient. People not deemed ill enough for admission were written prescriptions and sent home to their families.

Most patients approached the psychiatrist with deference but warmed to him as he joked with them. At the end of the assessment, some of the patients and their family members knelt in front of Dr Ajith, and with palms together, they touched the tip of their forehead, then bowed to the tip of his shoes. Sheepish, Ajith tut-tutted people back onto their feet. I was shocked to see this use of power and hierarchy.

Chamali explained that this practice is called 'worship'. Sinhala and Tamil children 'worship' their parents this way as a sign of respect and obedience, and patients worship the physician or anyone in authority as a sincere expression of respect and gratitude. I was ashamed. I had jumped to conclusions, seeing this as subservience.

On Wednesday afternoons, I attended the small outpatient health clinic adjacent to the psychiatric hospital. People arrived in rickety red government buses from miles away to have a mental health check-up and their prescriptions renewed. A doctor, Chamali and I listened to the progress report, most often given by a family member.

Chamali or the doctor interpreted for me. As I became comfortable with the process, I started asking my own assessment questions, offering information to facilitate diagnosis and treatment. I began to feel I was contributing something to the process.

On Tuesday afternoons and some Saturdays, I attended the Caregivers Society meetings and heard the narratives of parents and families, struggling to meet the needs of their mentally ill family member. During the meetings, a family member or a person with a mental illness stood, unannounced and sang a plaintive song in Sinhala or Tamil.

It was a touching, ancient form of communication, a song of profound grief and yet, a song of hope, soothing the patients and caregivers and arousing my own soul to kinship.

I was bombarded with stimuli all the time: visual differences, cultural differences and social differences. These differences, coupled with the cold weather and the language barrier, left me shaken and overwhelmed. I had to set limits on what was feasible to accomplish. There was so much work to do, and I realised I could not tackle everything.

Training took twice as long as expected, because everything that came out of my mouth had to be translated into Sinhala or Tamil. Pressure was building, until one day, as I rode home on my scooter, I could no longer endure the bumpy, muddy roads, the mist and the multitude of problems. I wept. My tears mingled with the raindrops as I made my way home.

Chapter 11
Life in the Freezing Cold

Longing for a warm fire does nothing to dispel the cold.

We were slowly adjusting to our new schedule and the rhythms of life in an unfamiliar environment. But there was one thing we weren't prepared for—the cold. In our new home, we nearly froze to death. We remembered that Upali had warned us, and we had assured him that it would not be cold for us, Canadians. However, it *was* very cold for us.

On most days, the temperature inside our home was about five degrees Celsius. Our breath was visible inside our home. It often seemed warmer outside in the rain than inside the house. Driving rain, propelled by fierce winds, blew in under the three-inch gap of the doorway.

The draft rattled the single-paned windows. Rivulets of condensation dribbled down the inside of the windowpane and puddled on the sills. We felt unable to bear the discomfort that seeped into our bodies and distracted us.

Each night, we crawled into our bed draped in damp sheets and damp bedding. Layers of fleece, socks and toques accompanied us to bed. A few weeks of experience provided a dismaying insight that this was not a temporary situation.

From the shops in town, we purchased several more wool blankets and layered them over the bed. We wrapped up in each other's arms and held on tight, hoping to warm the damp bedding. Whenever Bill shifted and wiggled, I commanded, "Stop moving around."

Like mummies we lay there, avoiding movement that created space for cold, damp air to whoosh in under the blankets. After about an hour of lying very still, a meagre heat built up inside the cocoon. Our neck muscles thawed, and we could fall asleep.

The damp seeped through the concrete flooring. Water dripped down the walls, leaving rusty-coloured stains. It was like living in a cave and I half wondered if stalactites were about to sprout from the ceiling. Rain trickled into the house via light fixtures mounted to the ceiling—drip, drip, drip.

The drips plunked into plastic buckets we had set out to catch the water and keep the tile floor dry. It was so slippery when wet.

Green mould grew like fur over my leather purse, the leather cover of my e-reader and along the back of our black, vinyl couch. Keeping down the green mould became a symbol of our misery. It was hard not to feel duped. We hadn't signed up for this. We began regretting our decision not to live in a yurt in Mongolia.

Each day, a small sigh of joy and a yelp could be heard from our tiny bathroom. Stripping for a shower and shivering, I stepped into the hot shower and stood under the streams of heat to soap up my hair with shampoo. "OOOOHM." The chant escaped from my slack lips.

Suddenly, cold water spurted from the showerhead and blasted my head. Cursing and shivering, I rinsed the foaming white shampoo, added conditioner to my hair and soaped and rinsed my body in the ice water that flowed over me. Stepping from the cold shower into an even colder room was a daily torture. I became skilled at showering quickly.

"Buck up, Wendy. You are tough. You will detach from this weather and this cold and the lack of hot water," I told myself. I knew I should be grateful, even for a trickle of hot water. "Shame on you," I scolded myself. We had what others in our village did not: running water in our bathroom.

Most of our neighbours had to use the communal washing facilities erected by the government. These facilities were often in the middle of the tea plantations or along the side of the main roads. The washing stations consisted of a concrete platform that had been constructed over a diverted stream.

This platform created a six-foot waterfall of freezing mountain water that cascaded down upon another platform where people stood to shower. These shower facilities had no walls or curtain for privacy. On my runs through the tea plantations, I often encountered someone bathing.

One day, furtive as a Peeping Tom, I saw a man washing his body by drawing his sarong up between his legs like a loin cloth, his hands inside the sarong, a gesture of modesty.

Sometimes as we hauled past private yards on the public bus or hiked through the tea plantation, I saw women bathing, shoulders bare, a colourful wrap covering their breasts and knees. I saw them reach up under the wrap and wash their private parts.

Sri Lankan women have long hair worn in long braids or twisted into a bun at the nape of their necks. Due to the weight of the hair, they need several rinses in the icy water to clean their tresses. On more than one occasion, I saw men lurking behind tea bushes watching the women, lust pooling in their eyes.

Every day, I passed people who had to fetch their own water. In the village, municipal water was pumped to standpipes around neighbourhoods. Villagers carried water containers on their bicycles or motorbikes to fill at the standpipe.

On my way to work, young boys balanced large water containers on the back of their bicycles, taking them home to their mothers before racing away to school. In the evening as I drove home, women and children filled buckets at the communal spigot for washing and cooking the next day.

I knew the weight of water. When my parents first purchased our lake property, they bought tiny trees from a local nursery in the hope that, one day, they would provide fruit to eat and shade from the hot summer sun. Unfortunately, the trees required more than rainwater to sustain them.

As children, my siblings and I were conscripted into water duty. Twice a day, morning and evening, it was our duty to haul cold water out of the lake into large white buckets. Immersing our bare feet into the cold water, we semi-filled two buckets and then we slogged the heavy buckets up the sloped and gravelled lakeshore to dump the water in the hollow at the base of the parched trees. It was hard work that left us flushed and panting.

This chore began on the first day at the lake in the spring and prevailed over the entire summer until autumn, when the weather cooled and the trees began shedding their leaves, signalling the return to school and relief from our water carrying. My siblings and I hated this seasonal chore, and we complained at the injustice of the hard work.

Yet, our Sri Lankan neighbours and their children hauled water every day, often twice per day and carried it for much longer distances than just up a short beach. They weren't watering trees for shade on a luxury property but drawing water for survival.

Through blogs, letters and Skype, we related the weather conditions to our family. Rather than expressing empathy, our family was amused that we shivered in the dark in Sri Lanka. What amused them most was that *Bill* shivered in the dark.

Bill was notorious for his worship of the sun and heat of the tropics. My family had watched Bill's growing excitement about living in a tropical country where, he believed, the sun's rays perpetually shone. But the sun did not shine in Nuwara Eliya. It rained.

The family's chortling and sniggering in delight from Canada could be heard all the way to the tiny island. Oh, they thought they were so funny. They had no idea of the damp and the misery and the mould.

We longed for our furnace at home that blew warm air through the heat ducts whenever the temperature dropped. We longed for our recliner chairs perched on either side of our gas fireplace. Reading in the evening, we flipped a switch on the wall and the gas flame whined then popped into an instant blue that warmed us.

I was disappointed in myself for longing for these comforts. I had thought I was strong and resilient and unspoiled, but I wasn't. I was selfish and miserable. But peering out our tiny kitchen window and over the concrete garden wall, I was reminded that the homes of our neighbours sat in mud. I felt so guilty.

Our home in Canada was beautiful and well equipped, and our apartment here had flaws, but many homes of our Tamil and Sinhala neighbours begged condemnation. Most homes sat on concrete foundations to ensure they did not slide away in the downpours, but many hillside country homes were corrugated metal shacks. The roofing material, held in place with large rocks and tree stumps, rattled in the biting wind.

Each day as I walked down the flight of stairs to our apartment, I looked over the wire fence that separated our yard from our neighbours' yard. I saw the home where an elderly woman and her very stooped husband lived. The tiny windows in their home were cracked.

Two of the windows that faced me were taped across with opaque plastic to shield the interior from the driving rain. Their front door hung ajar on one hinge. Blackish grey fire smoke oozed from under the eaves of the low roof. I also knew they didn't have running water. I felt shame at my weakness and grumbling.

We tried to find strategies to keep warm. Each morning, we closed the door to our tiny kitchen. We set water to boil on the stove. Boiling pots of water steamed up the tiny room creating rivulets of water down the panes of glass on the windows and warmed the kitchen. We dragged dining chairs into the kitchen and sat side by side, spooning down steaming bowls of oatmeal in the mornings.

Luckily, we had a gas range which simply needed a match to ignite the blue flame for cooking. More than 75% of Sri Lankans rely on firewood for fuel. As a precious commodity, wood was used only for cooking, not for heat.

Due to growing concerns about deforestation and illegal cutting of timber for fuel by villagers, it was forbidden to collect firewood in the forests except on Sundays. On Sundays, while we enjoyed an outing on our scooter, women dressed in faded saris, sometimes accompanied by a child of ten or twelve years of age, walked several kilometres to the forest. They needed to collect sufficient wood to last the entire week.

Entering the dense forests, hatchet in hand, they emerged several hours later with huge bundles of wood chopped in five-foot lengths. They carried the heavy wooden branches home on their heads. The children emerged from the forest balancing identical, but pint-sized bundles upon their small heads.

Women often worked in groups, and it appeared to me that they made the day a social gathering. They sat beside their bundles on the grass by the side of the road, drinking water from a flask and chewing on betel nuts that stained their teeth red. They seemed engaged in animated conversations. Then, break completed, they heaved the bundles upon their heads and followed the highway down the hill into their villages.

As we drove by on the scooter, fascinated by the size of the bundles, I compared their life of survival to our life of luxury and abundance.

All our complaining left us with a sense of shame. We had made a choice to volunteer. It was a temporary situation for us. We had made a commitment to VSO for two years, but we were not prisoners to that commitment; we were free to leave at any time.

People living in Nuwara Eliya had no choice. This was their Gama, their ancient village. This was the home of their ancestors, their birthplace. Families lived on the same plot of land for generations. Mobility was a difficult concept for Sri Lankan people to consider. Sri Lankans considered being separated from their Gama as a deep hardship, a type of grief.

I was beginning to understand this more and more over time as Bill and I began to grieve for Canada, our family and our warm home. We marvelled at the grit and resilience of the people living in the Nuwara Eliya mountain region. Day by day, like them, if we were to stay and work here, we had no choice but to endure the climate.

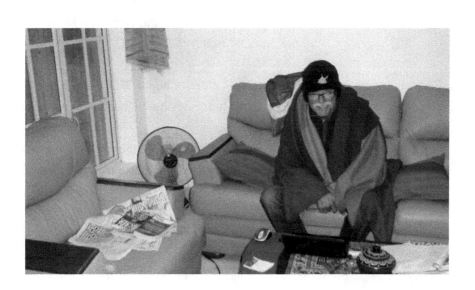

Chapter 12
Acculturating

I continued to compare and contrast, compare and contrast. I was driving myself crazy. So, I threw off the bonds of my culture and embraced the reality of the new and wonderful.

As the weeks went by, we started to feel more at home. Bill did not work in Nuwara Eliya, as VSO was unable to find him a position. Undaunted by his lack of work, Bill carved himself a position as a domestic.

In the market, he purchased two large plastic tubs. In the red tub, he soaked and scrubbed our clothes in hot soapy water. Then he transferred them into the large blue tub of cold rinse water. Over and over, he rinsed the clothing in the freezing water until the bubbles cleared.

On those glorious, rare days without rain, he hung T-shirts, pants, underwear and panties from the lines strung about the yard, pinning them with red and yellow plastic pegs. But most days, he had to sling clothes inside on a wire rack he had purchased from the market. Nothing dried. Some mornings found me gripping my electric hair dryer and blow-drying my clothes enough to wear them.

Bill's domesticity included shopping as well. With a list in hand, he entered the stores, which were reminiscent of mercantile stores in the 19th century. Every store, jammed from ceiling to floor, included a jumbled loft at the end of a staircase cluttered with pots and pans.

Stores sold everything and sold nothing: one type of comb, one type of bowl, one type of basket, one bolt of cloth, one type of shoe. No selection or choice existed. Bill moved along the cracked sidewalks from one cluttered store to another, putting off bargaining merchants, trying to locate an item he could then scratch from his list.

Balancing on the scooter, Bill carted home bundles, groceries, a printer and everything else he thought would be useful. Laughing, he recounted his market stories, often apologising for subpar purchases.

Bill made our dinner. I left my cold, damp office at the hospital and drove home in the cold rain to a warm pot of saeraiy (tasty) stir-fry and *rasneiy bhat* (hot rice). Hot comfort food always helped to quell the anxiety and tension.

Bill was a proud role model of domesticity and gender equality. Our backyard was like a fishbowl as neighbouring homes sat on higher ground. On some mornings when the sun did shine, our neighbours could see the 'Doctor lady' sitting in the sun enjoying her breakfast coffee, while the man of the house squeezed out the sheets and towels with his frozen hands and then pinned laundry on the clothesline.

I was a bit disappointed though. Other volunteers like Bill, for whom VSO had not found work, created work. A friend of ours found employment as a teacher at an international school in Colombo. Another volunteered for a women's centre after VSO found her husband a position but not one for her.

But Bill did not seem motivated to find work and wasn't hassling VSO to find something for him. He was alone a lot, stuck in a damp, cold house and not creating a meaningful opportunity for himself. I started to resent his lack of motivation.

"It's like he's on holiday," I groused to a friend at home one day. I struggled with the inequity of this arrangement. It wasn't supposed to be like this. We were supposed to be in this together.

My work at the hospital was stressful. I had to communicate with a vocabulary so limited it could be written on the back of a hockey card. I didn't get a rest in the afternoon, and I didn't get coffee on demand. In the meantime, I felt he was enjoying his life as if in vacation mode!

As a therapist, I know that anger can be an opportunity for introspection, discernment and change. I considered what was happening. I studied my feelings and realised why I was resentful. I was jealous. *I* wanted to be the domestic person.

"He doesn't do anything to make the home homey," I continued my grumbling to my friend at home. "I'd have planted a garden in the yard, decorated and put pictures on the walls."

"Didn't Bill work until he was sixty-eight years old?" My friend reminded me. "And didn't he work as a provincial court judge? Now he deserves a retirement."

I shifted my thinking by talking to God and about my feelings. "Wendy, isn't this what you wanted?" He asked. "I thought you wanted to do development work. I thought you wanted to work for me. Didn't you want to learn another language? Didn't you want to experience a different cultural context?"

"This was what I wanted, God," I mumbled back between breaths. "I was the one that applied to CUSO. I am doing what I wanted. Thank you, God." I praised Him for his wisdom and for his gift of opportunity.

I started to use a hymn as a cognitive strategy to offset my mood: "This is the day; this is the day that the Lord has made. Let us rejoice, let us rejoice and be glad in it."

As I processed my feelings, I began to reframe my thinking and noticed that his being home actually reduced my stress. I didn't have to worry about banking or going to the market. I didn't have to do housecleaning or laundry. I realised that supporting me to do volunteer development work was Bill's very noble contribution.

His support enabled me to persevere in the commitment of volunteering. Without it, I might have returned home early as some volunteers do who are unable to overcome the difficulties of climate, the work expectations, or the cultural adjustment necessary for a successful placement.

We were both elated when in February we welcomed our first house guest. Our VSO colleagues were reading our blog about the cold and becoming curious about Nuwara Eliya. One of our nearest VSO neighbours, Kamal, called to say she was coming for a visit from Kandy.

She arrived a few days before Bill's birthday. We ditched Bill. We wanted to purchase a sarong for him as a gift. A sarong is a length of plaid cotton fabric printed in red, yellow or blue and wrapped like a long skirt around the waist of the man. Kamal and I hit the stores, searching for a traditional sarong in batik, the sarong worn on formal occasions by the local men rather than the plainer tartan worn for everyday activities and fieldwork. We were becoming friends and I felt something ease within me.

In a crowded clothing store, we selected a sarong. It was teal blue with a batik border print. I had already scouted out a bakery where we could purchase a birthday cake. That night, Kamal, who was an excellent cook, created an Indian meal and we sang "Happy Birthday" to Bill. He was sixty-nine years old. It was glorious to have company and to be alive.

I purchased the sarong thinking that wearing one here in Sri Lanka would be a bit of a novelty and provide him with apparel for special cultural events. What I did not count on was his sheer joy in wearing the sarong. "It is comfortable, easy to tie, and I think it looks good with sandals," he said, admiring himself in the mirror. It felt strange to come home from work to find him doing the laundry or reading outside in his long skirt instead of his usual attire of trousers or shorts.

I decided to continue Sinhala lessons. I wanted to be able to communicate in the workplace. I learned from the landlord that Sandamali Koswattha, a woman about thirty years of age who lived across the lane from us, taught in the Magastotha Private English School. One morning, as I returned home after my early run, I bumped into her coming down the lane in her beautiful sari. She was on her way to the school.

Panting, I introduced myself. I inquired if she might be interested in teaching me Sinhala. She did not hesitate to insist on a price of 2500 rupees (about $18 CAD) for each lesson. I was happy to pay the demanded sum, and we agreed to do our two-hour lessons on Tuesday and Thursday evenings. So, twice a week, Sandamali left her crowded home across the muddy alley and marched down the twelve wet tiled stairs to our tiny apartment.

When it was time for the first lesson, I was nervous. As soon as she rapped on the door with militant authority, I swung it open. She stood in the dark drizzle bundled against the cold and damp.

She pushed past me to the dining room table where my little moleskin notebook that impersonated a Sinhala dictionary sat alongside my scribbler. The smell of turmeric and yellow curry swept in after her as she rustled about organising herself at the table.

She had created and brought worksheets which I was expected to complete. They included fill in the blank sentences, verbs with no endings and little cartoon pictures requiring me to write small sentences and phrases describing childlike events.

She wasted no time. "Naeae. Say it like this," Sandamali commanded, her dark brown eyes, crusted in black lashes, were glaring at me. "Naeae," she said louder. I stared at her mouth as she spoke. Her thick top lip curled back, baring her white teeth. From between her full, dusky lips a bright pink tongue protruded.

"Naeae," I intoned, trying to replicate the complicated sound, forcing my tongue, teeth and lips to match hers. It sounded like a horse's neigh.

"No! You can't speak Sinhala with your tongue inside your mouth. Stick out your tongue," she demanded. I could hear her frustration rising to match my incompetence. "Naeae," she demonstrated again, her tongue striping her chin.

"Naeae," I tried again, wanting to please. I stuck my tongue out as if my doctor were depressing it with a large flat Popsicle stick. It made me shiver thinking of the dry wooden texture of the stick pressed so near my gag reflex. I wiped my chin dry with the back of my hand.

"Hondai, good," Sandamali congratulated me. A pride of accomplishment mixed itself with a growing insight at the daunting task ahead. "You write Sinhala quite well," said Sandamali, offering a shard of hope.

The Sinhala alphabet was a series of swirls and curls formed into decorative letters. Each letter represented a sound. I could write and read simple Sinhala words reasonably well, but the sounds stumbling out from between my folded tongue and gritted teeth had no intelligible linkage to this curly alphabet.

"Say dakunata," she demanded.

"Dakunata," I repeated.

"No, dakunata." Her exasperation was audible. I looked at her lips and the protruding tongue. The *D* was actually a *Th*.

"Thakunata," I repeated, my tongue between my teeth, as if I was saying the *th* in 'thanks'.

"Hondai," she nodded. "Dakunata is the Sinhala word for 'right.' 'Dakunata haerenna' means to go right or turn right. 'Wamata haerenna' means to go left or turn left."

"Wamata," I repeated with some confidence.

"Wamata," she said in distain. I listened and looked at her mouth. She wasn't saying *w*amata, she was saying *vw*amata. It was as if the *V* and the *W* were combined, morphed into some fluid consonant non-existent in the English language. I pursed my lips into a *V* and then into an oval to make the *W* sound. She still didn't seem pleased with my attempts to mimic the language.

Over time, I deluded myself into believing that I was making progress, and I decided to practice on the trishaw driver who chauffeured me home from the marketplace. From the ripped black vinyl seat, I leaned forward and shouted, "Vwamata Haeraenna, Vijithapura by-road puluwan, left turn onto Vijithapura By-road, please."

"Mama English Naeae, I don't speak English," he said to me.

"Naeae, naeae English, no, not English," I hollered to make myself understood, amazed at his stupidity. Didn't he know I was speaking Sinhala? "Vwamata Hearaenna," I repeated, gesturing to the left.

"Ah, Vwamata Hearaenna," he repeated. He veered left just in time.

"Dakunata Haeraenna," I shouted to him to go right.

"Huh?" He shrugged and shifted the gears of the trishaw. He was close to passing the turn to my home.

"Dakunata Haeraenna," I screamed at him.

"Ah, Dakunata Haeraenna," he shouted back and careened right.

Sinhala was so hard, and the lessons seemed useless. Nobody understood a word I said. But Sandamali still demanded I learn and speak the language. I began dreading Tuesday and Thursday nights. Anxiety played havoc with my stomach.

I prayed a tiny novena, hoping for divine intervention. "Dear Lord, please don't let Sandamali come tonight for my Sinhala lesson." My novena flopped on His deaf ears. Sandamali never missed a lesson.

Twice a week she asked me in Sinhala, "Oyage something, something waedikaerannawa?" Twice a week she asked me this same question. And every time I stared at her without a clue of what she was asking. She chided me, "I ask this question every time I come to see you. Why don't you understand me?"

"I don't know why," I grovelled, head hanging in shame. "I just can't hear what you are saying. Please slow down."

"Naeae, I will not slow down. This is how people speak. You need to listen." My Sinhala lessons were torture.

Then one day, as I prepared for her arrival, I placed plain sugar cookies (biscuits, they are called by the Sinhalese) on a plate to accompany the hot milk tea Sandamali and I sipped during our lessons. As usual, Sandamali bustled in, settling herself at the table without fuss. She spied the cookies. Her eyes flashed to mine. I nodded towards the biscuits.

Sandamali relaxed. During the lesson her fingers slid across the table, snatching the biscuit as if expecting to be scolded. Bundled in her woollen hat with tiny purple flower motifs dotting the band, a thick black woollen muffler wound around her neck and a grey hoodie, she sat in my freezing home chomping on biscuits, sipping hot tea and teaching.

Treats of sweet cakes and cookies and milk tea became the key to our lessons. I stopped dreading my lessons. I think she had dreaded them too! We chatted in both English and Sinhala. She continued to correct my pronunciation, but we got used to each other's voices and accents.

Slowly but surely, the differences between us started melting. She relaxed her expectations of me, and I stopped trying to be perfect. She reduced my workload as I became more honest about my struggle with the translation at the hospital and began providing her with real examples. In turn, she used these examples to give me practical support to overcome the translation issues I encountered at work.

I stopped being the student and she stopped being the teacher. We moved from our rigid roles circumscribed by expectation to a more fluid place where learning shifted as needed. Truth and honesty began forming the basis of the relationship. Sandamali shared her financial worries.

Her shoulders slumped under the weight of supporting her parents, two of her aunts, her two teenage siblings, her husband and her one-year-old daughter. The family also relied on her to finance her brother's education as a physician, the family's ticket to financial security. However, his graduation was at least ten years away.

"My meagre teaching wages are the only reliable source of cash income," she confessed to me. Her family grew vegetables around the small plot of land the house stood upon while her husband earned some daily wages picking vegetables in season for local farmers to sell at the markets and roadside vegetable stands. The rupees I paid her for each two-hour lesson was not her slush fund. It was a survival fund.

"I am angry that I have to go to work and cannot care for my own small baby," she shared, tears welling in her luminous eyes. Her mother, sisters and aunts provided her childcare, but working outside the home deprived her of caring for her own child herself. She was envious of those at home and felt burdened by her imposed responsibilities. I had nothing to offer except empathy.

We shared a friendship based on reciprocity of mutual respect and genuine interest in each other. Sometimes we laughed and giggled like schoolgirls. Other times we grumbled at the shortcomings of our husbands. I asked her questions about culture, gender, fashion and politics.

I realised that learning about a culture was much more than language. I realised that issues of gender and motherhood bonded us while her poverty and my privilege polarised us. I offered her novelty from her drudgery, a chance to practice her English and most of all, some income and hope.

She offered me an education in Sinhala language and culture, but also through her, I was allowed a tiny peek into the circumstances of my neighbours who lived inside their rickety homes.

As my Sinhala started to improve, the trishaw drivers began to take direction from me in Sinhala. "Madame, you speak Sinhala?" one of them inquired in English, his eyebrows raised in disbelief.

"Oh, yes," I replied, lips pursed, teeth separated. "Mama Sinhala puluwan, I speak Sinhala."

"Hondai, good." The driver chuckled and pressed his dusty bare foot to the gas pedal.

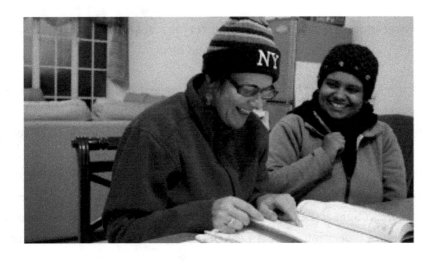

My Sinhala lessons with Sandamali

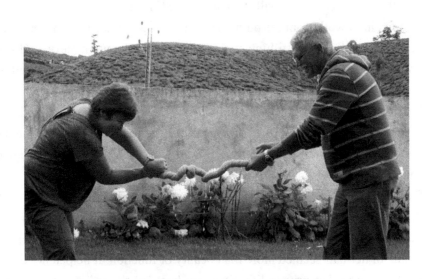

Bill and VSO volunteer Anne Murray wringing laundry

Chapter 13
Knocking Down the Barriers

Obstacles have a way of popping up, but the resourceful have a way of slithering around them.

As the weeks passed, my work began to take shape. I had to assess and draw a line on what was doable in the little time I had. I consulted with Chamali, who by now, had slipped into the role of being my translator. But she had become more.

She was my first Sri Lankan friend and my closest work colleague. I discussed all the assessed areas that we felt needed interventions. I explained the areas where I might assist but there were so many options. I threw my hands up and expressed indecision in a Sri Lankan term, "What to do, Chamali, what to do?"

She laid her tiny hand on my fleeced jacket and smiled, "First, we will move you into the clinic. Then, you will teach us, naeae?" I smiled at her. It was settled.

I settled in to work from the outpatient office. It was the old Lion Beer brew kitchen, with the fireplace still intact. Chamali arranged a work party, and with the Caregivers Society assisting us, we painted the entire place a warm yellow. It transformed the old brew kitchen into a functional clinic.

Less than five feet tall and weighing all of 90 pounds, it was Chamali who set the tone for the clinic. Her patients never saw her hair down during the day as it sat braided and wrapped several times around her head and pinned under her nursing cap.

Each day, at the end of her shift at 4:30 p.m. she removed her cap like a holy ritual, unbraided her hair, which hung to her feet and brushed it out in long strokes. Then she re-rolled it into a large chignon at the base of her thin neck. This ritual of her hair seemed more than beauty or function. It helped her divide her work life from her private life. She then boarded the red government bus outside the hospital and travelled home as a woman, not a nurse.

Chamali was a Sinhalese Buddhist. She prayed and meditated before her shift. In the morning when I arrived at eight o'clock, the clinic was filled with the smell of incense, the smoke curling up towards a picture of Buddha that hung above the incense pot. Jesus' picture was also there, along with Hindu gods, Vishnu and Ganesh. Chamali honoured the patients' different faiths by hanging pictures of various gods in the clinic.

Chamali was my primary translator, and when I conducted training workshops, she often translated five hours per day. She never complained. I articulated my worry as she translated on top of her regular nursing duties.

"Chamali, you have so much work to do here. Everyone relies on you. I am sorry that you must translate all day for me too."

"It's okay, Dr Windy," she always said. "We will do it. It is important. I will sleep tonight. I am okay. I am learning from you when I translate," she pointed out to me.

I realised she was my conduit to sustainability, a critical hallmark of development work. There was an aura of holiness that surrounded her. She embodied compassion, empathy and genuineness, not only to her patients but to everyone she encountered. It made her beloved to all.

She abhorred the hierarchy of the medical system, the hierarchy that pigeonholed her as 'only' a nurse and 'just' a woman. She knew the ropes and cleverly orchestrated ways to circumvent policy in service of a needy patient. Each day, she wound around the hospital wards making friends, greeting old colleagues and garnering favours for her patients and her staff.

Altruism seemed innate for her. On days when we had to visit the main hospital, as we wove between the grounds and operating theatre, the women's ward, the men's ward, the diabetic clinic, Chamali poked her nose into each place asking for cardboard. She collected bits and pieces from packing that had once wrapped a doctor's chair, boxes that had once held paper, along with scraps of packing Styrofoam. These she lugged over to the mental health clinic and piled it in a corner.

One day, a very thin, shy young man dressed in worn pants and shirt arrived at the clinic asking to see Nurse Chamali. I called Chamali to the door. She bowed to him and bid him to follow her. She led him to the pile of cardboard and Styrofoam, then slipped him a few rupees as he departed the clinic, carrying the cardboard high above his head.

"Why did you give that man the cardboard?" I asked, confused. "I thought you were saving it for floor mats to absorb water when the patients arrived dripping wet from the rain."

"That man is a patient at our clinic, and one day he told me of the severe overcrowding in his home and that he is sleeping on the ground. He told me he was very cold at night, and that his weight was dropping, and that he was unable to sleep. I told him to come back in two weeks and I would have some cardboard saved for him."

"I saw you give him rupees. How come?"

"He needed the money so he could ride the trishaw home instead of walking with his shame. Everyone knows that cardboard is for people who do not have a bed." I felt ashamed of my lack of charity. I was freezing at night in my solid home in a bed with a mattress and with wool blankets piled high, expensive woollen clothes and snuggled next to another human being.

How did people endure this life? How did Chamali live here with such good cheer and such goodness? She became my role model.

I realised that Chamali focused on others, not herself. When the cleaning staff arrived to clean the clinic, she prepared tea, often rushing to a food stall to purchase savoury donuts called *ulundu vadai* while the kettle boiled. She returned with the donuts wrapped in newsprint.

She offered the cleaning staff a place to sit, and while they sipped tea and chewed on their donuts, she laughed and joked with them. While the rest of the hospital staff were not kind to the cleaning staff, Chamali always made them feel important and valued.

Besides Chamali, in our office, I worked with Karune and Mulkanthi. Karune, our clinic aid was a Sinhalese Buddhist about forty years of age, who spoke no English. He commuted each day to the hospital from Welimada, a community located along a horrendous strip of highway, often plagued with killer mudslides.

His smile and goodness matched Chamali's. Mulkanthi was also a Sinhalese woman, married to a Muslim Tamil, so she spoke Tamil as well as Sinhala and a tiny bit of English. She was our orderly for the clinic, assisting Chamali with medications, charting and translation of Tamil.

We became a strong team. I asked them to not call me Dr Wendy and insisted they call me Wendy, which they began doing. They were my colleagues, but they were becoming my friends. I felt less and less alone at the hospital.

Most of the general and psychiatric hospital staff was Sinhalese while most of our patients were Tamil-speaking. We overcame our language differences through gesture, expression and laughter. As we sat between patients or during unscheduled clinic hours, this team of comrades taught each other about languages, culture and some of our customs.

They taught me hospital politics, how patient care is managed and how to make do with little. Paper and pens were at a premium, so I learned to make notes on tiny scraps of paper from bins that we scrounged from the medical side of the hospital.

Chamali and I decided it was best to focus on teaching the doctors, nurses, hospital aides and community workers and to include the tea estate aides who worked on the plantations as health liaison people. We chose to teach the bio-psychosocial approach to mental health, which was current best practice in the West. This approach could assist in increasing a knowledge base, reduce stigma and increase the skills sets of doctors and nurses. Also, it was sustainable, an important marker of success for development work.

Stigma was tackled first. Throughout the assessment period, I discovered a distasteful haughtiness and blaming attitude of some of the hospital staff as if the mentally ill person or the family was somehow responsible for the illness. The key to reducing the stigma, I believed, was in creating empathy and unconditional positive regard for each person.

I began my first group training with the hospital psychiatric staff. In Ajith's office, we moved the desk aside and placed chairs around a whiteboard and projector. We began at eight o'clock each morning after the staff had arrived to work.

I had worked hard on a curriculum. My teaching style was Socratic; asking questions that provoke thought rather than memorisation. I began by asking the question, "Are we born equal?"

Hands went up. "Yes," said one nurse.

I pointed to another hand and nodded. The student rose, "I think that we are not born equal." Others seemed unsure, and a discussion ensued.

"If we are fortunate to be born with intelligence, are we equal to the person born with average or below average intelligence?" I asked. The class agreed that those with intelligence learn better and faster than others and can garner seats in universities and obtain high-paying professions.

"Did one person earn their intelligence or were they just gifted it from birth?" I asked. There was agreement from students that people did not earn their innate intelligence and so no fault could be placed on the less intelligent.

"If we are born with beauty, are we equal to those born ugly?" Students got it. They agreed that the beautiful are more likely to be selected for prestigious marriages and selected for jobs over equally educated and qualified candidates. "And if we are born into a wealthy family, are we more likely to get ahead?" I asked.

"Yes," they agreed.

"Did the person born into a wealthy family do anything to deserve or earn this privilege?"

"No."

"What about someone who had a loving family? Were they more likely to succeed than an orphan whose parents had died and was placed in an orphanage? What about the country into which you are born?" I asked.

"Do you think I was more likely to succeed just because I was born in Canada than someone born in Sri Lanka? Did I do anything to earn the fact that I was born in Canada?" People agreed I had done nothing to earn that privilege.

I pressed further, poking into something I had noticed in Sri Lanka. "Weren't fairer skinned Sri Lankans more likely to succeed than black skinned Sri Lankans?" They twittered. I had struck a chord.

Still lecturing, I shared a story. One day, on an excursion to Kandy, Bill and I rode the wobbly red train. Packed in amongst large shopping bags and cardboard boxes sat a Sinhala woman with her two children. The woman was friendly, using her elder daughter to translate for her.

As we conversed in a mixture of Sinhala and English, she unwrapped a package on her lap and extracted some lumpy peanut brittle. After the children each had selected a chunk, she offered some to Bill and me along with withered apples she pulled from a small basket on the floor. We nibbled at the peanut brittle as we lumbered along in the train.

Her older daughter was about sixteen years of age and was an exceptional beauty. I noticed a dignity and poise about her as well. I told the woman her daughter was very beautiful.

"Naeae, she is too black," she stated, wrinkling her nose in resignation as if nature had dealt the entire family a lethal blow. To prove her point, she began rubbing her daughter's forearm and pointing out the colour of her skin. The daughter avoided my eyes.

I was dismayed and protested that her skin colour did not matter. But it *did* matter to them. White was still better than black. Colonialism raged on.

I carried this discussion of privilege further. I asked, "If someone was born into a majority Sinhala family, are they more privileged in Sri Lanka than a minority Tamil? How does caste limit opportunity?"

I remember an instance from my own social work training when internalising this message of privilege left me ashamed. One of my first assignments during my social work studies had been about values. Writing my essay, I shared how, despite being on welfare due to my divorce, I was not like 'those people' on welfare. I was not one of 'them'.

My children were clean and groomed. I didn't drink and smoke. I managed the little money I had and had been able to avoid debt. My situation was temporary, I asserted in my paper. I shared my shame about being in the welfare office to collect a cheque with tattooed women and their dirty babies. I had different values than 'they' did.

A few days later, my professor waved me into her office to review my paper. Certain it was an A paper, maybe one worthy of publication, I perched on the proffered chair. She began berating me, "How dare you compare yourself to those you see in the welfare office? What makes you think that you are better than others who need welfare?"

I looked at her, confused. "You have been handed life on a silver platter," she said. I was on welfare. It didn't feel like a silver platter to me. I blustered, trying to defend myself, feeling attacked.

Softening in the face of my shock and anger, my professor explained to me, "Wendy, you have been given great intelligence and beauty. You are strong and healthy. You were born into a family that loved you and nurtured you and taught you to be resourceful. You were given a personality that is outgoing, but also tenacious and determined. Not everyone was gifted with these strengths out of the gate. Not everyone was nurtured."

I got it. My judgments shrank as my sense of remorse and shame grew. I rewrote the essay. The new essay acknowledged my privilege and fortune, my strengths and my good family of origin. I saw people differently after that. I saw oppression, injustice, lack of opportunity and success through a different lens.

The point I made to my students was that privilege exists, and once we understand that we have not worked for privilege, we begin to understand we have some responsibility to level the playing field for the others: the ill, the disabled, the developmentally delayed and a lower caste. It is the role of the privileged to assist the oppressed to topple injustices.

I knew I was shaking the tree at the foundations of our cultures. It was my hope that by discussing these issues in a safe, comfortable and supportive environment, a value shift might take place, allowing the nurses to view their patients with more empathy, understanding and less blame. I instructed nurses on the importance of unconditional positive regard, no matter the patient's culture, colour, caste, or position in society.

I set up role-plays to assess how they would respond to a patient. One nurse in role-play was asked to play the part of a caregiver and the other the role of a nurse.

"I am so tired and don't think I can go on looking after him," the caregiver lamented.

"Oh, no, don't say that. He needs you," counselled the nurse in role-play.

I instructed them, "By giving advice and not responding to the person's actual words and feelings, we negate their feelings." I asked them to consider the feeling behind the statements. One nurse said, "I think she is feeling fear." I taught them to summarise the problem.

Another nurse put it beautifully. "I can see you are worn out and tired, and you are worried you can't go on looking after him. Is that right?"

I taught students how to attend to the needs of their clients without robbing the client of their own innate problem-solving abilities. I also taught students to find the strengths in their clients and help them use that to work through their problems.

"You have been through so much in the past and you have overcome the problems. What have you done in the past that has worked to alleviate your strain? Is there someone you can ask for help?"

I taught students basic skills to ensure they elicited the entire story and to help them parcel out the problems into manageable chunks to better assist with an intervention. "You have told me so many things. Which of these things are troubling you the most?"

I picked away at the notion of hierarchy. Doctors were revered, and nurses seemed to have no sense of their own value in the nursing of the mentally ill. I pinned up a picture of a troupe of circus performers holding a star performer who was balancing precariously at the top of the human pyramid. I asked them which circus performer was most important in the picture.

"They all are," they agreed. They began to value their role and appreciate the importance of a team to serve the client or patient. Although they agreed with the concept of teamwork, they laughed at the notion of the actual application of equality in a team environment.

Hierarchy seemed entrenched in the society. People aspired to higher positions and felt the right to dominate others was earned. I couldn't help but wonder if this attitude was instilled by colonialism.

One day, when I was in the main hospital, the hospital matron in charge of all nursing approached me. The matron wore a navy uniform with a white apron tied at her back with a large nursing hat on her head that looked more like a nun's habit. She was seen striding about the hospital issuing edicts or sitting regally at her monstrous desk approving nursing leaves.

However, on this particular day, she approached timidly. "Madam Dr, we have heard about your training and my nurses also want your training. This is possible?"

I was thrilled. Rather than being viewed as controversial, the training was resonating, at least with the nurses. I was convinced I was on the right track. About twenty-five medical nurses attended the lectures over the next twenty weeks. We role-played in English and Sinhala and Tamil. We laughed hysterically as we watched each other practice, make mistakes and then hone the skills in simulated situations.

Before leaving Canada, I purchased a new Sony webcam and enrolled in a week-long, but intensive film school on Vancouver Island. This camera, along with the filming and editing knowledge gleaned that week, came in handy as I filmed the students practicing their skills. I even produced a small movie which highlighted their skill development.

Pirating some Sinhala music from the Internet, I set the movie to music and in the credit section, I showcased all the nurses' names. Chamali and I hatched a plan to demonstrate the skills to the doctors, psychiatrists and matron in a formal graduation ceremony.

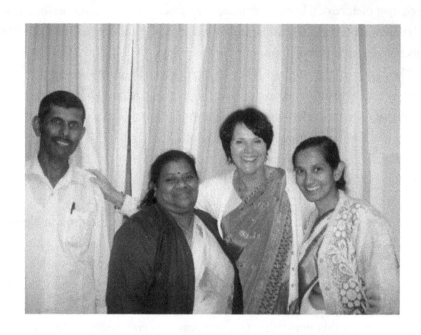

General Hospital Nuwara Eliya Mental Health Clinic Staff:
Karune, Mulkanthi, myself and Chamali. We made a fine team.

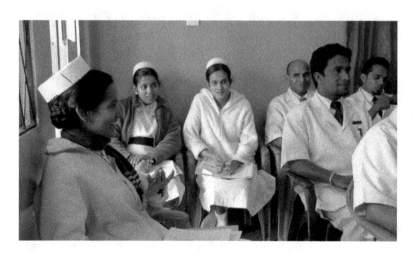

Chamali and I teaching the mental health course to psychiatric nursing staff
at the General Hospital in Nuwara Eliya

Chapter 14
Undressing at the Hospital

Nothing is so attractive as a person who can laugh at themself.

Sri Lankan women wear saris. A sari is a length of fabric about 9 yards long and four feet wide. Some women in Sri Lanka will wear western clothing or tailored blouses with tiered skirts, but professional women almost exclusively wear a sari. I wanted a sari to surprise the nurses on their graduation day and besides, they were so beautiful.

"I want to buy a sari," I explained to the Sinhalese shopkeeper as I peered into the doorway of his crowded and colourful sari shop.

"Ow, Madame," he replied with a flourish, luring me deeper into the store. "We have this cloth, Madame, it is silk." The salesman enunciated his English as he deftly layered several yards of peacock blue fabric across the counter. I shook my head and stuck my tongue out across my teeth to form the negative sound.

"Naeae, too blue," I said.

The salesman plucked another sari from a clear plastic casing and flung it upon the counter, "Or, Madame, what about this colour, like a sweet mango?" He trailed his weathered hand along the mango/orange coloured fabric with a bright pomegranate bordered fabric.

"Naeae, naeae," I gaped at the array of colours upon his shelves, my eyes searching for a colour that would resonate with my conventional tastes.

"This, Madame will like," he said, scooping a gold leafed ruby fabric from its plastic sleeve.

"Naeae, too red, something plainer," I said, exposing my lack of flair and convention. From under layers of brilliant colours, a gem gleamed at me. "That one," I said, pointing.

The salesman handed me the package, wrinkling his nose in admonishment. "This one, Madame? It is an old colour, not so nice." My fingertips sensed the silk spun by millions of silkworms. I smoothed the cloth and the fabric rustled like the leaves of a jack fruit tree in the warm breeze. The cloth was tan coloured, a silk blend with blue, green and apricot accents.

"I will take this one." Shrugging and sulking at my poor choice, the salesman proceeded to find his tape measure.

Sari fabric is sold in a long length of cloth allowing for one end to be cut off and sewn into a tight filling sari blouse that is more of a short bodice. The short blouse leaves the woman's belly exposed. The other end is used for the wrapping. It consists of one long continuous bolt of fabric, which encircles the waist several times and continues to the pallu, the bright and bordered end of the material that is draped over the left shoulder. The salesman, ancient measuring tape in hand, measured me for the sari blouse: upper arm circumference, bust dimension, length from collarbone to midriff. He appeared most careful with his measurements.

"This will be ready in two days," he said as he wrote out the sales slip by hand, passing the bill to a cashier. When it was ready, my little Nokia phone rang. "Madame, your sari blouse is ready for you to pick up," the salesman purred into the scratchy receiver. Bill, my trusty errand boy, jumped on our Scooter and raced to town to pick up the blouse.

I tried on the blouse in the privacy of my home. First, I put it on backwards, thinking the row of tiny buttons belonged in the back. "Shoot," I said, struggling out of the tight blouse. I was still sticky from the cold rain that drenched me on the way home from the hospital after work. I tried it on front ways.

I stuffed my arms into the short, capped sleeves. The cuff encircled my upper arm like a vice grip, forcing the fat of my arm to bulge out below the cuff. My thick upper arms resembled canoe paddles. I felt claustrophobic and trapped inside the blouse, not sure if the vice grip on my arms would loosen enough to set me free of the garment.

"Oh no!" Dismayed, I looked closer at myself in the mirror. The darts stitched into the blouse sharpened my breasts into cone shaped points, like a little girl playing dress up with pointy ice cream cones under her T-shirt. I was a Canadian woman and we had specialty bra shops to ensure our foundation garments formed us—rounded and full. "I am not okay with this," I moaned to no one as I looked down at myself. The scoop of the neckline was so low, that it revealed my bra and cleavage.

"Bill, come here and look at this," I hollered from the bathroom where I stood in front of the mirror. Bill gawked at my breasts, amusement twitching at his lips. I was not amused at his amusement. "You must come with me to the store when I speak with the tailor. This is too low and I am not going to show it to him without you there," I insisted.

So, the next day, we sped off to the Sari Shop. Half a dozen salesmen were loitering about the shop, waiting for customers and leaning in to listen as I explained the problems with the blouse. The man, who was neither the original salesman nor the tailor, suggested I try it on and show him the problem. The other salesmen drew nearer to the change room. Arms akimbo, Bill stood guard outside the curtained closet.

I entered the tiny, curtained change room, donned the vice grip blouse and stuck my head out from behind the grubby curtain. Clutching the curtain to cover my chest, I asserted myself to the group of men hovering outside the curtain, "I will show this to *one* of you. Just one of you can come in here and look at this." I knew I was shouting.

A man named Jude was appointed to inspect the problem. He entered the change room drawing the curtain across the opening. He turned and faced me in the tiny cubicle. He looked down. He assessed my snow-white pointy breasts tumbling out of the skimpy blouse. Shifting his eyes away, he stared at the wall of the closet. Raising a straight pin, he fumbled. He didn't know where to pin and he didn't know where to touch.

"Madame, there is a problem. There is a problem with this sari blouse," he agreed, backing out against the curtain, cheeks blazing. My cheeks blazed too.

Then, Jude explained, in Sinhala, to the salesmen lurking outside the curtained room that there was a serious problem with the blouse. They conferred in Sinhala to the best course of action. Nodding in consensus, Jude telephoned Amar, the man who had taken the original measurements, on his cell phone. "You must come. Madame's blouse hondai naeae (no good)." Amar had just stepped out for his lunchtime packet of rice and curry when he received this urgent summons to return.

Soon Amar appeared, panting and wiping his mouth with the back of his hand. He was hustled to the change room where Madame was standing. He poked his head past the curtain. A puff of curry wafted about the tiny space.

"This is no problem, Madame. No problem at all. Look, we will just do this, and we will do that, and we need to bring it in here and here." Touch, touch, pat, pat. "Yes, yes, too pointy, you want it smooth, naeae?"

"Ow, I replied, face turned to the side, unwilling to meet his gaze. I pointed out how tight the cuff was on the upper arm. "Normal, normal" he indicated, nodding in understanding.

The tucks and pleats were successful. The arm cuffs were widened to accommodate my paddles. When I picked up the blouse a few days later, the blouse fit and covered my bosom.

The morning of the graduation, I wrapped myself in the Sari according to the instructions of the salesman. It took at least an hour. I had tucked in everything and the garment seemed secure. I studied my effort, "Not an unreasonable first attempt," I congratulated myself while pirouetting in front of the mirror, smoothing lumpy pleats.

I rustled out the front door, sat side-saddle on my scooter and bumped along the rough road to the hospital. I entered the auditorium where the graduation was to take place. Nadie and Sister, two of the nurses in my training were already there, preparing the room. They gawked at me. They had no idea I was planning to wear a sari.

"Ooh, aww, Dr Windy, you wear a sari today," they exclaimed in surprise and delight, fussing over the sari. Then they became concerned, "Hmm, tsk, tsk, naeae, naeae" they shook their heads, turning me about as they examined the wrapping job. "We will wrap you," they determined, pulling at my garment. Here?" I asked, mortified. We were in the main auditorium of the hospital.

They unwound the wrapping, muttering at my failings. I had the fabric inside out. They set that right. As they peeled the last wrap from around my body, they discovered my thong underwear. I hadn't planned on revealing my knickers that day. They giggled and twittered at my unusual foundation garment, making comments in Sinhala that I did not understand. One comment I did understand.

"Sudu noona" (white woman), they giggled as they examined my fleshy, dimpled and very white buttocks. Brown hands patted my bum. "No underskirt, Dr Windy?" Nadie asked in shock.

"No, I didn't know I needed one," I moaned, mortified that my bum was hanging out in the cold in the hospital auditorium near the open doorway. Jude, the salesman, had failed to mention an underskirt. The nurses were innovative. Nadia produced some surgical gauze and Sister cut a strip sufficient in length to wrap and tie around my waist. A bundle of safety pins and a card of straight pins were produced. Nadia and Sister folded and pleated, draped and pinned me until I had on a very comfortable, well-wrapped and beautiful sari.

I still had to pick up the projector from the mental health clinic, so I headed out of the auditorium. The sari was a bit tight around my ankles forcing me to mince down the hallway of the hospital. Out on the hospital grounds, needing speed to cross the distance to our mental health clinic, I grabbed the pleated fabric at the front of the dress and lifted it high enough for striding. Chamali, who accompanied me, chided, "No, No, Windy, just pinch a small amount of the sari, just an inch or so." She demonstrated, plucking up a small pleat and lifting the hem a half inch, just so the toes of her sandals were revealed. I had received my lessons in being lady-like—lankawa style. I again slowed to a snail's pace.

Mincing again, I swayed back to the auditorium with the projector. In the auditorium, I found the nurses blowing up red and orange balloons and awaiting the film debut. The guests arrived.

Standing at the podium, I welcomed everyone and explained the bio-psychosocial approach to mental illness, the value and utility of interpersonal skills for patient interaction, and the hard work the nurses put into learning the new skills. After dimming the lights, the amateur show I had filmed and directed flickered across the screen. The nurses sat with glowing faces, watching themselves and their colleagues on the big screen. They finally believed they had important new skills to better communicate with their patients.

Dr Ajith and the matron congratulated them and handed out certificates of completion that I had had approved by the Sri Lankan Ministry of Health. Only certificates recognised by the Sinhala government were deemed valuable for adding to a resume. The formal portion of the ceremony completed, we consumed the sweet *kiri bat*, then the doctors and other guests exited the auditorium.

Then, mischievous Chamali played back the movie with the embedded music and turned up the volume. Tossing balloons up into the air, my students began giggling and swaying to the music. It felt unbecoming and childlike to be tossing balloons to music in the workplace.

My pretence glared me in the face. Was I uptight or were they childlike? My cultural norms, and perhaps personality, were uncomfortable in the face of their playfulness.

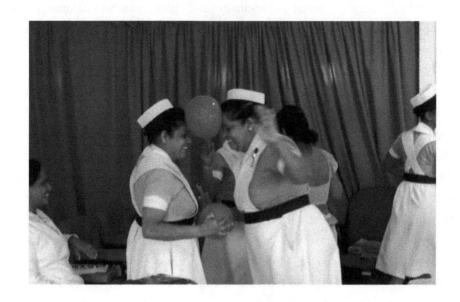

Graduating nurses horsing around with balloons

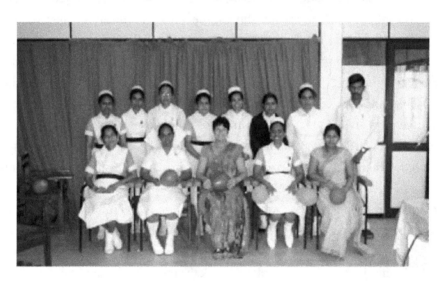

First group of general nursing staff graduates from the mental health course

Chapter 15
Close Encounters with Locals
Unique Traditions, Unique Habits

I felt a bit like a tea bag dropped into boiling water inside a tea pot. I was
steeping in a culture.

April is 'Spring Season' in Nuwara Eliya. It is the one month of the year that the weather is likely to be hospitable. The average annual temperature in Nuwara Eliya is 16 degrees Celsius with 1905 millimetres of rain per year. But in April, the rain becomes intermittent and the weather warms. Families escaping the smouldering heat and humidity of Colombo flock to Nuwara Eliya.

Free of the intense heat of Colombo, they snuggled in the hotel beds with a loved one, giggling under the blankets, enjoying the novelty of trying to generate warmth. For some of the wealthier families in Colombo, Spring Season is an annual family tradition, and it coincides with Sri Lankan New Years.

The Tamil New Year (Puthandu) and the Sinhala New Year (Aluth Avurundu) are celebrated between 12th and 15th April. One Monday in April, all the doctors I worked with came crowding into our small clinic. Something was up. They stood in a line and with folded hands, bowed low to me.

"Happy New Year, Wendy," they said in Sinhala as they straightened and shook my hand. I was so touched. I was appreciative of the thoughtful gesture. I mirrored their bow of affection. "Happy New Year to you all, too."

To celebrate the New Year, Wednesday, Thursday and Friday were official government holidays. Bill and I took advantage of this leave time and hopped a bus to head south. The bus descended from the tea plantations in chilly Hill Country down through the rice paddies in the southern interior towards Hambantota, a city along the east coast of Sri Lanka.

From Hambantota, we followed the coast where the weather warmed, and the bus filled at each stop. The salty smell of the ocean became seductive. We ended our seven-hour-long journey in Tangalle, and the Lonely Planet guidebook directed us to Ganesh Gardens. It was sheer heaven with its swaying palms, beautiful beach, good food and cabañas.

We visited the towns of Matara and Mirissa. We booked a whale watching tour and we read good books. We suntanned and we swam. We met and played board games with an American couple working at the American Embassy in Colombo.

One morning, we arose and left Ganesh Gardens to exercise before the day became too warm for walking. We ducked under the low swaying palms as we left the tiny beach resort with its bungalows half buried in white sand. On the rutty, dusty, rocky road, we dodged insolent water buffalo, huge hissing monitor lizards and defiant cows that mooed as we edged past them.

We noticed that the cows had been branded. We stopped and stared in disbelief and revulsion at the curling strips of flesh dangling from their sides. It was horrible. Hot iron branding is illegal in Sri Lanka, but some farmers, fearing theft and distrustful of ear tagging, continue to use this method. Unable to fathom the pain the creatures must be in, we hurried on our way.

People greeted us from their homes along the rough path. Some people sat in green plastic chairs, and some stood in the doorways, waving as we passed. One house was so close to the road that when the woman leaned out of her window, her head was right above us. She called out to us, "Ayubowan, hello," and invited us in for tea.

Bill and I were wary. We didn't invite strangers walking by our house in for tea. Her invitation made us uncomfortable. Each day, as we walked the path, this woman and her family invited us for tea. On the third day, sitting on green lawn chairs outside their home, they called, "Hello, where are you going?"

"Just for a walk," I responded with a smile, not engaging.

"Come for tea, madame, sir," said the older woman. I kept walking, but Bill hesitated.

"Yes, please come into our home for tea," said one of the younger women, taking advantage of Bill's hesitation. They were so insistent that I stopped and turned back, catching Bill's eye and nodding at him.

"Okay, we will come for tea," I agreed, dragging my feet towards the home. Bill was surprised at my change of heart, but game as always, he accompanied me inside. The Amma (mother) introduced her four adult children, her teenage boy and her two grandchildren. One by one, as they were introduced, they embraced us and kissed each side of our cheeks.

The adult girls hustled off into the kitchen and returned with trays of delicious milk tea served in chipped English teacups along with many types of commercially prepared cakes and desserts. I worried at the cost of those biscuits. A bundle of small bright yellow bananas perched in the middle of one tray.

It felt a bit weird, all of us just smiling at each other. We pinched the small handle of the teacup as we sipped on the sweet tea. The boy in his early twenties, dressed in a yellow T-shirt and brown shorts, broke the awkward silence.

"We had a tsunami, a giant wave," he explained. "On 26 December 2004. None of my family was killed or injured, but our home was destroyed." He pointed to a place closer to the water where there remained a small pile of rubble. "We had this new home built through the help of a British aid organisation. We are very lucky."

This new home, situated in a dusty dirt yard, was surrounded with banana palm. It was small and constructed with rough grey cinder block. The living room was long and narrow and filled with plastic lawn chairs. The home had a smooth concrete floor. There was no glass in the windows.

"We are still very frightened that the wave will return," the boy told us. His family nodded in agreement.

One of the adult daughters spoke. Tiny and frail looking, her timid smile belied the weariness in her eyes. "I work as a cleaning lady at the hospital, while my brother works part time at the hotel where you stay. The others cannot find work," she stated. Her younger brother nodded in agreement.

"I want to go to Saudi Arabia to find work," interjected the oldest daughter, about forty years of age. "I must make enough money for a dowry so that I can marry."

The mother coloured. Bowing her head, she confessed, "My husband takes the drink, so we have not been able to save money to marry our daughters." The husband was not in the home, but the family pointed to a small, identical home next door which he occupied alone. The British NGO had provided two homes on the same property to protect the family from the emotional and financial effects of the father's alcohol abuse.

Despite our cultural differences, the family exuded warmth, amiability and a sense of fun. We thanked them for inviting us. They invited us back that evening for a New Year's Party. We declined. They invited us back for tea the next day. We said we'd see. They all kissed us again.

After four days of rest and relaxation in the tropical paradise, we did stop in at their home on our way out of town to say goodbye. We were kissed again and the Taata (Dad) of the clan was over for a visit this time. He kissed us too. We expected him to ask for money. He didn't. Shame tweaked me for being so sceptical of their intentions.

We headed into Mirissa to catch the bus for the long ride home. Before boarding the ancient bus, we milled around Mirissa's colourful downtown, killing time. I spied a blue sign in a dusty office window. The red and white lettering read: "Dr (Mrs) S. Soundararaja."

These Victorian era handles hang from medical shingles all about the country. Bill and I expressed dismay that empowered female physicians were compelled to hang out their shingles with names listing their marital status. "You should list your name like that, now that we live here," Bill said with a grin. "You should be Dr Mrs Wendy Blair," he joshed.

In Mirissa, Bill braved the bus station washroom, so I sat alone on the bus depot bench. As I waited for him, a middle-aged woman in a blue sari plunked herself down beside me. She eyed me up and down. I smiled and turned away from her stares.

Undeterred, she leaned into my shoulder. "Where are you going?" she asked me. By then, I understood this commonplace inquiry translates as, "How are you?"

"To Nuwara Eliya," I replied, shifting my seat slightly. She moved in a little closer and looked into my eyes.

"Oyage bandala innawadh, are you married?"

I nodded, biting into a ripe plum I had purchased from a fruit vendor near the station. She nodded in relief. I dug in my pack and offered her a plum.

"Thank you, Madame, Mrs," she said, biting into it. We sat in on the bench munching our plums as Bill came sauntering towards us.

"My husband," I said, identifying Bill. Pleased at this evidence of my marital status, she shuffled over to make room on the bench for him.

We boarded the bus at 7:30 a.m., and with a groan, the bus surged down the highway. We were packed like sardines; every space on the bus filled with a package, an elbow or a knee. The conductor instructed us to move into the middle of the bus, but there was nowhere to go.

The bus was jammed, yet it continued to stop for more passengers who flagged it to a stop. The conductor kept hollering at us to move deeper into the bus.

Flustered, I leaned into the body of the person in front of me and pressed with some force, my leg against the man's leg. He was forced to shift an inch. My opportunistic foot thrust its way into that space while I began to lean in and apply pressure with my hips and shoulders against the man's back. To avoid toppling all the people ahead of him in a domino effect, he had to shift his feet again.

My other foot found the gap. Pressing my hips into the man's bum and then spooning him, I inched along. Each move required an anchor point. The grab bar, which extended from the luggage rack above the seats, stabilised me as I inched along. Bill crept along behind me using a similar technique.

We weren't the only aggressors. At times, I had a man's elbow threatening to take out my eye while my hip was pressed into a short man's stomach. Another person would embark, and everyone would shift again. I'd have my breast pinned against a woman's shoulder and my butt against a seated man's cheek. With each body shift, the combinations of interlocking body parts shifted.

The bus capacity was fifty-five seats. We were close to one hundred people for most of the trip not counting the cargo of leeks, carrots, baby carriages, parcels and duffle bags that had to be stored somewhere by the conductor. He is the man who takes the fare and grabs the sack of corncobs from a passenger struggling up the stairs of the bus and shoves it under the seats.

He settles the smelling sack of onions beneath the feet of a passenger and slings the boxes tied with string up front and gestures for the passenger to take his seat upon the boxes. Into crooks and crannies of the bus, including the passengers' precious leg and feet room, he bundles, heaves, shoves and crams goods and cases and sacks. He also ensures the bus stops at the destination of the passengers and fetches the correct parcels that he has stored somewhere in the bus.

Our conductor was about thirty-five years old, organised, efficient and objective as to who got a seat or not. He handled the chaos inside the bus with a steady hand. However, his judgment became severely impaired as he continued to allow people carrying huge bundles to board that took up more space than the people. Suddenly, he was behind me.

"Madame," he said, apologetically asking for permission to proceed down the length of the bus to collect the fares. I nodded and tried to make space for him to proceed. However, there was no give in the walls of people that surrounded me. Undaunted, he pushed and pressed and turned, slowly morphing into a space.

He arched his hip towards me as he moved into the tiny space. We were face to face in a deep pelvic lock, our thighs crushing into each other's groins. Our eyes locked in fear. Then, in humiliation, our eyes unlocked, desperately casting around to look anywhere but at each other.

We began struggling and writhing. The hip lock was bolted shut. Aghast, Bill grabbed my right arm, yanking me towards him as a shocked male passenger began pushing the conductor in the opposite direction to dislodge the vice. The other passengers sat riveted by the unusual situation.

The wall of people morphed again, releasing the guy to press forward on his mission to collect more fares. My cheeks flamed. I buried my face into the armpit of my husband. I imagined smirks but instead heard women clucking in sympathy.

I avoided looking at the conductor for the rest of the journey and in turn, he avoided me. However, my shame soon turned to anger at the dangerous overcrowding, discomfort and lack of safety standards the government of Sri Lanka imposed upon their people.

The journey's difficulties continued as the loaded bus edged its way up the mountainside. The rain was incessant. The narrow, muddy shoulder of the road was riveted with washouts. The back fender of the bus scraped the road as we veered around a corner featuring a one-thousand-foot ravine. From the bird's eye view within the bus, it appeared as though the balding tires were going to slide into the abyss.

I wasn't the only person in discomfort. A young girl, about ten years of age, who seemed to be travelling alone, worked open her rusty window and half-standing, vomited out of the window. She wiped her mouth with the back of her hand and then vomited again. She sat down, looking straight ahead. We sighed in grim relief as the bus edged into its stall in Nuwara Eliya's bustling bus station.

We arrived home to some mail from the VSO. I tore it open immediately. "What the hell?" I exclaimed, thrusting the letter at Bill. VSO had continued to apply for a visa to relocate me to Jaffna and in the envelope were government visa re-application documents we had to sign. To my horror, my name was inked into the forms as "Dr Mrs Wendy Nordick." There I was. A woman identified by her marital status.

Spring season was over. After April, tourists flee Nuwara Eliya in droves as the temperature drops. The inevitable cold rain and damp sets in again, the mist obscuring the mountains. A shivering groan could be heard from inside our home as Bill layered back up in fleece.

After returning to work the next Monday, my stomach began grumbling, and I had to dash to the bathroom. I had a bout of diarrhoea. My bottom glued to the toilet, I stared at the toilet paper dispenser. Unlike most train stations and restaurants, the hospital supplied toilet paper, but this time, the roll stood empty, the grey cardboard tube rebuking my unpreparedness.

I was going to have to use the spray hose. Some bathrooms, including the hospital and our home, provided a hose with a nozzle near the toilets. It looked like a garden hose. A Sri Lankan bidet.

This is what is to be used to clean up following a bowel movement instead of toilet paper. I had never used it before. Bill, on the other hand, was quite handy with the toilet hose.

"I like the freshwater method," he exclaimed one day, emerging from our bathroom. "It is a much cleaner way than wiping," he claimed. "I'm not depositing all that needless toilet paper into the environment either." He looked smug. However, I had not witnessed his cleaning process, and he had refused to give me hosing lessons.

I hovered over the toilet for so long my thighs had begun to burn. My aim was off that day, and I had already peed on my shoe. *Crap.* I grabbed the black hose, twisted my body around and aimed the nozzle at my bottom.

As I pressed the button, water shot from the nozzle, spraying and splattering all up the back of me and into my dropped drawers. The cement floor was soaked. *Crap.* Mortified, I searched the bathroom with my eyes. There were no rags or hand towels. A toilet plunger mocked me from the corner.

I pulled up my dripping drawers that had chilled to the point of freezing then I hosed the pee off my feet. I squared my shoulders. With the dignity of a queen, I emerged from the bathroom in wet, beige pants. Smiling, I sidled past Mulkanthi and Karune, betrayed by my squishy wet sandals and the dark footprints following me on the floor.

I remained hunched at my desk, busy with paperwork and shivering from the cold until quitting time. The next morning, I stuffed a roll of toilet paper in my purse, stashed a couple of rolls in my office and bought a large package for the hospital bathroom.

In May, Vesak celebrations took place around the country. Vesak is the holiest of Buddhist religious celebrations symbolising the birth, enlightenment and death of Lord Buddha. Having lived in Canada, historically a Judeo-Christian country, the rituals of Buddhism and other religions outside of Christianity were unfamiliar to me.

Long before the actual day of Vesak, I noticed an expectation of joy, hope and celebration in the air. In the clinic and around our neighbourhood, I overheard talk of fasting, cooking and feasting. In the week before Vesak, the usual decorum that greeted me as I entered the hospital was interrupted by an artistic eruption.

People were sitting on the floor and tying sticks together to build frames for their paper lanterns. Their hands were busy gluing and cutting coloured paper. In the clinic, we made our own lantern. Karune constructed the frame, and Mulkanthi chopped up bright coloured shapes from crepe paper and made rainbow-coloured streamers. Chamali and I glued flower designs into place.

The beauty and variety of the lanterns was not realised until the actual festival. At nightfall on Vesak, the lanterns were lit and hung everywhere. Every shop on Main Street featured a beautiful array of hanging lanterns. It was mesmerising to behold.

Lanterns, aglow with lights, floated on ponds like giant water lilies. They hung, festooned in coloured paper and soft white lights from homes, telephone poles, police stations and government buildings. Schoolyards and temples sailed these beauties in the wind. Lanterns twinkled, exuding light and hope everywhere.

What struck me was the sense of joy, peace and belonging that was apparent in those who participated in the celebration. It was a religious celebration, but it was also much more than that. It was a time of creativity, ritual and tradition. It was a time for family. It was a time for personal reflection.

Perhaps religion is the vehicle for spiritual events where we can come together to share and belong. Vesak reminded me of Christmas, and I felt homesick.

Our remedy for homesickness was to travel. Transportation in Sri Lanka is like placing your head on a guillotine block and never being quite sure if the axeman will show up. It is frightening. However, we gulped and placed blind faith in a bus or train that, in our country, would have been towed to a salvage yard.

After work, the Friday following Vesak, we rushed to catch the five o'clock bus to Kandy for the weekend. We hailed a trishaw, jumped in and sped off down the hill towards the train station in Hawa Eliya. About a kilometre down the road, the little red trishaw spluttered and died. The driver explained to Bill, "The problem is in the motor, sir."

Hopping out, we hailed the next trishaw whizzing by. We hopped in and without further delay were transported to the train station, where we learned that first-class was sold out, so we purchased second-class tickets. At the station, we both headed to the toilet.

The first and second-class ladies' room on the train platform was a yellow stained squatter toilet. Faeces, splattered about by some sick passenger, had decorated the walls. Toilet paper was non-existent. I straddled the bowl and planted my feet on the wet and slimy latticed footstalls and relieved myself.

A sign above the sink read: *Please refrain from washing feet here*. I doubted I could get my foot into the sink. Bill reported to me the men's urinal bowl was broken, so he had to take careful aim to keep his shoes dry.

We awaited the train on Platform One. Finally, a red and brown train arrived. Only then did we realise that the train to which we were entrusting our life was constructed in the colonial era with no refurbishing in the past two hundred years. As we climbed aboard, we prayed that at least the braking mechanisms had received attention since Victorian times.

Bill and I stood on the shiny metal platform between the cars, peering inside to locate our seat. Unbeknownst to us, this relic of a train had been scooping up passengers all along the route from further south, so by the time it rattled into Nuwara Eliya, there were no available seats. There was no available cargo space either. We stood in the doorway of the train car, but as more passengers crowded on board along the route, we were pressed deeper and deeper into the centre of the car.

Large windows on either side of the train were thrown wide open to manage the growing humidity. Men dangled outside the open doorways, carrying on conversations through the windows to passengers inside the train. Kids hung their arms out the windows only pulling them inside in the nick of time as the train careened near a tree or a cliff.

115

One ingenious lad made a kite from a plastic grocery bag and a bit of string, and he sailed it alongside the train as we whipped around mountain tops, through tea plantations, past long waterfalls, across wide trestles that straddled deep canyons and through tiny villages.

A seated family of five took pity on us and offered up their seats on a temporary basis. They helped us stow our huge knapsacks that blocked vendors selling waeDi (snacks) from pushing past us to garner a sale. The alternate sitting and standing as we traded places with the family provided relief for us all.

A musician blew a harmonica while his partner drummed on a bongo drum. Three men sang along. Our homesickness was dissipating.

Once in Kandy, we hailed a trishaw to take us to our hotel. The little blue trishaw trundled up the road a mere five hundred meters and died. The driver twisted in his seat to look at us and stated, "It is out of gas, that is the problem. Just wait, we get gas there."

He pointed to some vague location. "You stay," he instructed. He hopped out and began pushing his trishaw, with us still in it, towards a petrol station not yet visible. He pushed and pushed and then exclaimed in shock, "Oh, my Gowd! My pants!"

I looked over. In his effort to push, his pants had slid off to his knees. He was so embarrassed. Yanking up his drawers, he resumed pushing his trishaw towards the petrol station. Bill had jumped out to help him.

"Oh, my Gowd!" The guy's pants had slid off again! He stopped the trishaw and looking at me whilst fastening his pants, he said, "It is the button, Madame. That is the problem." We were hysterical.

We made it to the petrol station. The man wiped his sweating brow, filled his gas tank and we were again on our way to the hotel. He was a good sport and happy to supply us all with a good laugh. Tipping him, Bill encouraged, "Buy yourself a good belt with this!" Chuckling, the man pocketed the money and drove off.

That evening, we climbed the hill to where a Giant Buddha looks out across the valley to the Temple of the Tooth. This temple allegedly houses Buddha's tooth. We gazed at colourful homes clinging to the lush green mountainside. Roofs of red tile glowed in the warmth.

Kandy Lake gleamed in the valley, surrounded by mangrove, palm and giant Bodhi trees. The leafy palm treetops sang with birdsongs and monkey hoots. In the warm breeze, the trees swayed, making a soothing rustle. The view from the

Buddha took our breath away. You could feel and smell the ancient, the cinnamon and cloves, and the exotic. It was miraculous. We explored the entire weekend.

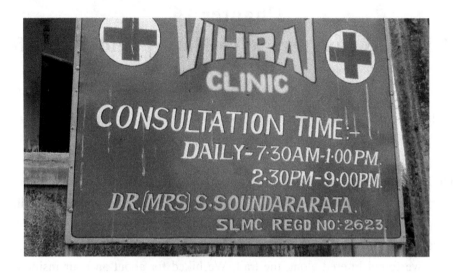

Marital and gender declaration that irked me

Chapter 16
Close Encounters with Nature and Wildlife

At first, nature can astound, disgust and frighten but then, with exposure, it bores, delights and befriends us.

On Easter Saturday, and it being a dry day, Bill and I set off to explore the forest that bordered the tea estate near our home. We stumbled onto a footpath leading deep into the forest. The trail was discernible for the most part, but where it became obscure or divided, we marked it with branches, sticks, rocks or plastic bags we found littered along the trail. We hiked for about an hour inside the forest, and when the trail became too obscure, we turned back for home.

Once home, and puttering about, Bill hollered out to me, "What the hell? Come and look at this."

A shiny black creature, about two inches long was moving across the tiled floor. It looked a bit like a slug but had a different snout; it was more like a proboscis. It seemed to use the snout not only as an appendage but also to sense things.

It was weird! We wondered what kind of creature it was. Bill, his hand encased in tissue paper, plucked it up and threw it outside.

About fifteen minutes later, Bill hollered again, "One of us is bleeding. There is blood all over the floor."

Sure enough, blood tracked into the bedroom and kitchen. We both still had our thick wool hiking socks on. Bill stripped off his socks. He looked in horror at his feet. Black leeches clung to his feet and ankles. He was bleeding from four sites on his feet. Horrified, I stripped off my socks and sure enough, I had three bites that were bleeding away, and one leech was still attached.

Bill tried flushing a leech down the toilet, but this most resilient and fascinating creature swam with strength in the current of the flush and attached its upper body to the slippery porcelain; and swung its lower body up and attached it, then swung the lower part forward, end over end, just like walking.

It was bizarre. Bill fished it out of the toilet and squished it. I used a shoe to squish another one. As their bodies popped, the blood sucked from our feet squirted out all over the cement of the outdoor patio.

By now, we were disturbed by this invasion. Stripping down, I shuddered as I tugged a leech off my outer upper thigh. I had blood everywhere inside my pants. Now frantic, we stripped down to nothing and examined all the nooks and crannies of each other's body to ensure no creatures had nested.

I inspected our hiking boots and not finding any, I concluded we had rounded them all up until…I realised I had one attached to my baby finger. I screamed as I flung the leech across the room. That night in bed, things were moving. We felt leeches everywhere. Probably we sensed that we would soon meet them again.

One long weekend, Marjorie, a VSO from Colombo, Bill and I decided to hike the Knuckles Range. Knuckles Range is situated between the Kandy and Matale Districts in the interior of the country. It is a UNESCO heritage site due to the endemic flora and fauna. It is often touted as a top attraction in tourist pamphlets. We had been anxious to see the Knuckles and needed a good long, therapeutic hike.

Marjorie left Colombo by boarding a bus to meet us in Kandy. We had dinner in a nearby guesthouse and retired early. The tour began the next morning in a 4x4 safari Jeep. The jeep took us to the trailhead where we hiked five hours into camp.

Here, we had our second confrontation with leeches—hundreds of them! Our guide, Amul, used pure Deet on his bare feet but for his clients, he carried a mixture of Dettol and water in a large green spray bottle and every hour or so soaked our socks and boots. Marjorie concluded that leeches had evolved to know that Dettol meant human beings and believed they are *attracted* to it.

She may have been right, as these bizarre and disgusting creatures seemed undeterred by Dettol. We bled all over the place. To my great horror and disgust, one ventured up my shorts to bite my unmentionable nether region, which my travelling companions found amusing.

Initially, Marjorie and I screamed when we found a leech attached to us. We tried scraping them off with rocks and sticks but the numbers multiplied. Bill dug out his Leatherman and used the pliers to pick them off for us. However, due to the sheer abundance and tenacity of the leeches, we began plucking them off with our bare fingers and flinging them as far as we could, only to find them inching their way back to our feet.

They littered the one-hour stretch of the hike known as Leech Lane. As we walked along, we could see the small proboscises of the leeches poking up from the ground like budding plants, sensing our arrival. In terror, we raced through this part of the hike. Stopping on the trail meant certain invasion.

In our haste, Bill had a couple of rough stumbles, one a direct face plant resulting in broken eyeglasses and a broken cell phone and a backwards fall into a foot of water soaking a lush paddy field. Marjorie reframed his first stumble as, "Elegant slide, Bill," his next slip down a slope as, "Good lead with the bottom," and then, "Fancy footwork," when he recovered from crashing into the weeds along the path.

Luckily, Bill received no serious injuries, just minor bruises. However, I was stung by poison nettle. Although invisible, these stings left my legs burning and itchy. This condition, along with potential boils, can last for up to a month. Luckily, my stings settled after a few hours.

Knuckles Range is spectacular and rugged. It lies in the most remote regions of Sri Lanka and is unspoiled and raw, serene and quiet, like the hush of a whispered prayer. The mountains are littered with ancient villages of approximately ten families each; these villages hug the steep cliffs or lie deep in lush jungle amidst emerald green paddy fields.

We saw huge grasshoppers and giant spiders lying in wait for prey in their webs. Birds fluttered about, monkeys peered out from tree branches and we were fortunate to see a rare snout-nosed horned lizard laying her eggs.

Butterflies flitted everywhere. Sri Lanka has two hundred forty-four species of butterflies of which twenty-three species are endemic to Sri Lanka. We watched the mating dance of a huge pair of black and white common Mormons. The air was electric with cicadas; their deafening cries came in regular, systematic sounds, like the crashing of an ocean wave upon the shore. We sniffed wild cardamom and wild nutmeg.

On the second night, we bunked down in caves. These ancient caves are still used by people harvesting cardamom and by the toddy tappers, who harvest the palms to make liquor. During the day, we traipsed through pygmy and bamboo forests.

We splashed in waterfall pools populated with freshwater crabs and tiny minnows. We dined on rice and curry for breakfast, lunch and supper. I, as usual, maintained a huge appetite, while Marjorie and Bill gagged down enough to keep nourished.

One of the porters, clad in flip flops, ambled ahead and swung his machete carving out a trail allowing us to proceed through the thick overgrowth. He chopped bamboo canes and handed us walking sticks. We couldn't have managed without them. It was hard slugging for four days.

Our knees hurt by day two and by day three, we were all on Ibuprofen. We were struck by the way some others had to make a living, and discussing that one night with Marjorie, we realised she was becoming a dear friend.

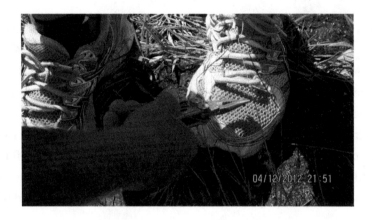

Bill pulling leeches out of my shoes with his Leatherman

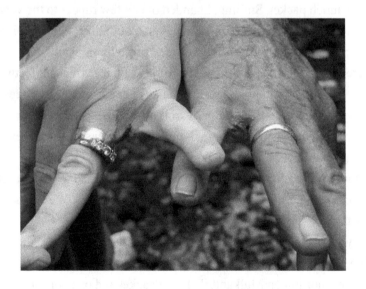

Matching Wedding Ring Leech Bites

Chapter 17
Bonding over Insects and Barbed Wire

Food is the medium that miraculously transforms a stranger to a beloved.

Chamali, Mulkanthi and I ate lunch together each day at the clinic. I had been bringing my own measly lunch derived of spicy chickpea crackers and cheese, but Chamali recommended buying the lunch packets sold in the stalls on the hospital grounds. The food in the lunch packet consisted of a cup of rice, a vegetable curry, meat or protein curry like soybean and some sambal for spice.

This food was placed in portions upon a plastic wrap, which was then twisted over the food. Then the whole bundle was placed in old newspaper and wrapped again.

Each day, I grabbed my umbrella and hurried down towards the stalls and selected my lunch packet. Smiling, I handed over a few rupees to the vendor who grinned with gapped teeth poking from his mouth like uneven piano keys. Poverty deprived people of the ability to seek orthodontic work.

Children everywhere are at the mercy of how their permanent teeth grow in, sometimes resulting in gaps, bucked or uneven teeth or missing teeth. Often people in the west rectify these dental variations with expensive dentistry. Here, however, the uniqueness of an original, unadjusted grin sometimes resulted in a charm that was at once captivating and becoming to me.

Clutching the lunch packet against my body, I returned to the unused office in the clinic where we ate our lunch. Mulkanthi made us tea. We spread our food out on the table.

"Oh, you have soya curry," remarked Chamali and without asking permission, she proceeded to divide my curry into three equal portions. Then, she placed one portion on Mulkanthi's lunch packet and one portion on her own. I had one portion of soya curry left on my packet. She dispersed some of her *seeni sambal* to our packets and divided Mulkanthi's potato curry and dispatched portions of it to her packet and mine.

This distribution of food was a cultural practice. Then we sat, bundled in our woollens, mixing the food with our fingers, blending the flavours to perfection before making a mashed ball and pressing it into our mouths. We talked about our families and our cultures. We spoke about our work. We gossiped and we laughed.

One day, Chamali blocked me at the doorway to the clinic. "Windy, don't buy food from that vendor where you buy your lunch. He has a bad reputation," she declared, wrinkling her nose in disgust. She recommended another food stall for me.

I complied and began purchasing my lunch packets from the other vendor. However, a few weeks later, Chamali announced that I was not to buy any more lunch packets from any of the stalls on the hospital grounds. She declared that from then on, she and Mulkanthi would be providing me with lunch.

"Why?" I asked, puzzled. Silence greeted me. "I don't understand."

Chamali and Mulkanthi crowded close to me. Chamali looked around to make sure there were no eavesdroppers and whispered to me, "Windy, we didn't want to tell you, but one day when we shared food from your lunch packet, I found an insect." Chamali's head bobbled in disgust. I wanted to vomit.

"That is why I told you to change the place you bought your lunch packet," she explained. Then, she and Mulkanthi moved in even closer to me, our heads touching.

"But look what we found in your lunch packet today." Bewildered, I stood there waiting, unsure what she will show me. Her hand fled to the pocket on her nursing uniform and fished something out. It was a twisted piece of barbed wire! Mulkanthi and Chamali nodded their heads in satisfaction that I now understood their concern.

"That is why we will make you lunch from now on," Chamali stated. They stood firm, and I didn't want to disagree. I loved their food and didn't enjoy thinking about biting into a cockroach or a piece of barbed wire. However, I was not going to let these ladies with limited income provide my lunch.

We negotiated a deal. Chamali and Mulkanthi would bring the curries that they made each morning before work, and I would purchase a rice cooker from the shops and supply the rice which we would make fresh each day in the clinic.

That weekend, I purchased a rice cooker and some rice. The next Monday, we topped up the rice cooker with plain rice and water and plugged it into the outlet on the wall. Then, to my surprise, with a nervous giggle, Chamali placed the cooker into a deep drawer in a metal filing cabinet while the rice steamed.

I didn't understand why, but she didn't want Dr Ajith to find out we were cooking in the clinic. We all twittered at this conspiracy, especially when Ajith stepped into the room shortly afterwards. We worried about the smell, but he did not seem to notice. This became our lunchtime ritual and was a dear time of friendship and belonging.

Chapter 18
Ups and Downs at the Hospital

I always plan for the inevitable, but the inevitable never appears as I expect. It always seems to take a different form.

Work ramped up. The more I taught, the more work I seemed to generate. On the days I taught the nurses in the hospital auditorium or on the ward, I would grab my umbrella and trundle over the soggy brown hospital grounds to the Ministry of Health building to procure the projector I needed to display my computer presentation. An eight-foot chain link fence surrounded the building, which forced me to pick my way through the mud all the way around to reach the main entrance.

Up two flights of stairs, I looked for Samij, the man who was responsible for all the audio-visual equipment for the Ministry of Health in our region. Despite phoning ahead to reserve the equipment, I always seemed to be a surprise to him when I showed up.

Although eager to assist me, he dashed from room to room, fetching the projector, digging through a drawer here and there and fumbling through desks and cupboards in search of a working cord. Handing over the equipment, he always asked me, "How long do you need this projector, Doctor?" He guarded that projector as if it was a solid gold bar.

"Until about three o'clock," I reported looking straight into his eyes, trying to convince him of my honesty.

"Very well, Dr Madame. But you must bring it back here at that time. You must give it to me. I am responsible."

"Ow, Ow," I agreed, bobbling my head in Sri Lankan body language.

After several instances of me returning undamaged equipment, I felt somewhat offended by the routine of the instructions and the distrust. He trusted no one, it seemed. I learned later that due to high unemployment, a government job was a coveted prize. The security, the wages and the retirement pensions compelled people to follow rigorous workplace procedures.

One day when I was returning the equipment, another man, Mani, approached me, asking me what I was doing over at the hospital. After explaining my mental health teaching position to him, he insisted that I needed to do some lecturing at the Ministry of Health office as well. "We know nothing. We need to know something," he pleaded bobbing his head.

That afternoon, I asked Chamali about what the Ministry of Health might need in terms of instruction. She told me that the Ministry of Health office was the meeting place of the public health inspectors (PHIs), child protection workers (CPWs), family workers, addiction workers and family violence workers who met once a week to coordinate services.

I realised there was a definite need for linkage between the hospital and the community support system. At that time, once a patient was discharged, there was very little community support. Even medication regimes often fell apart due to the distance from a doctor.

Travel was often too onerous in terms of cost, travel time, means of transportation and expense of accommodation. Many discharged patients required a caregiver to assist them, thus doubling the expense. A further systemic problem was that there were few avenues for the community to access a psychiatrist in any proactive way in order to avoid hospital admission.

I agreed to teach the community. I was not sure if I had anything to offer them but if they desired learning about the bio-psychosocial model of mental health, then I reckoned, I might be of some assistance. I went back to find Mani and asked him, "Can you arrange for Chamali and me to attend the next meeting of the Community Group? We will need to assess their needs. It is important."

He agreed, and we were invited to speak. After introducing Chamali and myself, we advised them of our work at the hospital. We then spent the next two hours examining the complexity and service gaps in community mental health issues and how mental illness, addiction, forensics, family violence, child protection, nutrition and poverty affected people and how to develop greater reciprocity and linkage between the hospital and the community.

This group of people were practicing social work by western standards but had no specialised training in any of these fields. All the same, they were intelligent, dedicated, experienced and had found many community solutions.

I needed funding to run this training session, so at the next Provincial Ministry of Health Meeting held in Kandy, I made a presentation and received funding from the regional district to run a mental health course for community social service workers.

Chamali and I decided to first run the already developed curriculum on the bio-psychosocial aspects of mental illness and to assist the community workers, and the community itself, to overcome some of the stigma and stereotypes often applied to the mentally ill. Before long, I was delivering the lectures, and Chamali volunteered to translate.

One lecture focused on teaching how to conduct a mental status exam. This exam is performed by a practitioner on a patient by examining them under categories such as appearance, attitude, behaviour, mood, thought process, insight, judgment and so on. I taught the components and descriptors within each of these categories and then needed to teach the class how to apply the information.

To add some levity and interest to the next session, I enlisted the help of Bill, who was willing for any diversion by this time. We planned a role-play, and I wrote a bit of a script for him. Chamali chortled all week about the pending spoof.

I told the class a foreign man had been admitted to the psychiatric ward and that, for the purpose of education for the community group, I was going to bring him to the Ministry Office the following week to conduct an interview in their presence. The class assignment was to listen to the interview and to conduct a mental status exam using the components and descriptors they had been taught. Bill's alias was Delusional Billy.

Billy believed he was a gem miner and that his brother and his wife were stealing gems from his mine. I introduced him to the class and then, with his consent, I interviewed him while the class listened. He was dishevelled, paranoid somewhat belligerent, and he believed that leeches were attacking his legs.

or than I had realised. Chamali and I could hardly
oled anyone but they enjoyed the application
of August, these thirteen community social
my Community Mental Health Course.
, that comes from teaching. I always felt so
sion. I saw the students applying the knowledge
their new and useful practice tools. Yet, the

exhilaration was often followed by bouts of exhaustion. Teaching took a toll on me.

As I continued to teach, I started preparing Chamali to co-teach the mental health awareness course I had developed. Sustainability is a hallmark of effective development work. It was my hope that once I left, Chamali would have the skills and knowledge to teach the course herself, in her language, without the need of a translator.

She had already been through the course as translator/student four times and was well versed in the content. In anticipation of teaching, she re-wrote the presentation slides in Sinhala. When the hospital requested another session of the mental health course, we were ready and co-taught the course.

Near the end of September, Chamali taught the mental health course to tea estate health workers on her own. I was very proud of her as I sat at the back of the class, not understanding a single word, but confident she was passing along all her learning. She was lovely to watch in her quiet, confident, humorous manner.

In the clinic, we worked so seamlessly together that sometimes I forgot that she was translating and used the time to assess the reactions in the patient as she spoke. After each session, Chamali instructed me in cultural aspects that impinged upon the patient's situation, thus shaping my own understanding of the complexity of the problem.

We learned from each other. Our relationship was one of reciprocity and mutual respect.

I had started another project. I was still appalled that our patients at the psychiatric ward sat on their bed, day in and day out, with no mental stimulation or attempts to improve their function. I had to do something.

I knew that Marjorie was an occupational therapist, so I sought and received permission and funding from VSO to have her come to Nuwara Eliya and run a workshop for the psychiatric staff. Chamali agreed to translate again.

Marjorie stayed with Bill and I in our little house for the weekend. On Monday morning, she swung her leg over the back of my scooter and hung onto my waist as we set off in the rain, past the wet racetrack, towards the tattered hospital.

Marjorie taught the attending nurses and support staff the theory importance of stimulation and activity for patients with mental entertained us all with her own brand of hilarious humour. In the afternoon, she led the psychiatric staff onto the open ward and modelled games and activities.

In a version of musical chairs, Marjorie had all patients and staff stand in a circle with a chair for everyone, except one person. She explained that we had to shout the name of a fruit, in English or Sinhala, as we threw the ball to a person across. But if she shouted "mango," everyone had to take a seat.

There was much hilarity, and some catatonic patients perked. Then, she produced bongo drums, and one of the support staff played the drums. He broke into song and the patients danced about the ward.

Crayons and paper became the focus of another activity. Marjorie asked patients to draw their home and the people who lived there. Once completed, Marjorie had each patient speak about his or her own family. It was informative not only from a 'get to know them' perspective, but also from an assessment perspective.

Marjorie assisted the staff in overcoming some of the biases held about the patients: the staff could see that the patients were human beings with a family, hopes and dreams. It was an emotional day for me. I felt privileged to have a colleague like Marjorie and to know that I had been instrumental in some joy for the patients and some learning for the staff.

I decided to apply for more funding. Through a grant from the European Union, I was able to purchase plastic tables for artwork and for eating. At the local furniture store, I purchased lawn chairs for the ward, so patients didn't have to sit on their beds. I bought nail polish and hand cream for the ladies for some self-care and beauty, and bought stacks of coloured paper, safety scissors, tape, blank paper, coloured pens and crayons.

I purchased cheap musical instruments and badminton rackets, horticultural tools and plants with which to develop vocational skills. I purchased plastic storage containers to hold the supplies. I gave these supplies to the head nurse. I created a schedule of activity to be used on the ward and the nurses nodded as I presented the schedule and pasted it to the wall with felt markers to indicate when the activities had taken place.

A week or so later, I went to the ward to check on the progress. The tables and chairs had disappeared. Patients were sitting on their beds again, looking vacant. The chart was untouched. I was upset and tracked down the head nurse.

"Where are the tables and chairs we bought for the patients?" I asked standing with my hands on my hips, looking him in the eye.

"They are locked up, Doctor. The patients will just steal them."

"No," I insisted. "The tables and chairs were purchased for the patients, and they are to remain on the ward. Now, let's get some help and put them back," I directed.

"Ow, Doctor." The nurse fished around in his pocket and produced a key. He walked to a closet situated just off the ward, inserted the key, and swung open the door. There sat the plastic tables and chairs. The tables had the legs removed for easier storage.

"Now, what about the schedule?" I asked. "I see that nobody is following up on the activities. Why not?"

"Dr Madame, the paper will be all gone, and the patients will steal the colouring pens. I am accountable for everything, and if we let the patients use them, then I will be in trouble."

"Why is ball not being played, why are the patients not doing agriculture, why is there no music?"

He shrugged. "The nurses do not like to do the activities," he reported.

That afternoon, I spoke to Dr Ajith. I explained the issue, and to my surprise, he also just shrugged and laughed. "They are worried the patients will steal."

"Doctor," I spoke with authority, "you have the power and authority here on the ward. Will you speak to them about the tables and chairs and insist they perform the activities on the ward as part of their job?" He bobbled.

Two days later, I returned to the ward. The tables and chairs were again missing. The schedule remained untouched. I stomped into Ajith's office and insisted he speak to his staff. He bobbled.

I felt very confused and frustrated. Chamali tried to explain that the staff feared that they would be fired if something went missing from the ward. I let it go, for the time being. I was teaching so much that I had little time to be fighting over tables or nagging nurses to do their job. But somehow, I felt they didn't value the effort it took to secure Marjorie, and it felt like the work to obtain funding for the equipment was futile.

However, with some shame, this incident made me realise that I might have made a mistake in my development work. Development must be bottom up, with ideas and suggestions bubbling up from the grassroots of the community or organisation.

I had sat and discussed with the nurses the value of Marjorie coming and the importance of activities on the ward, and they had seemed to be excited about it, but I believe they didn't realise that I was not going to be running the activities each day. I had assumed that they would be glad to implement the scheduled activities. Apparently, they weren't.

I tucked this into my hat and vowed to not let this happen again. I would be very clear next time.

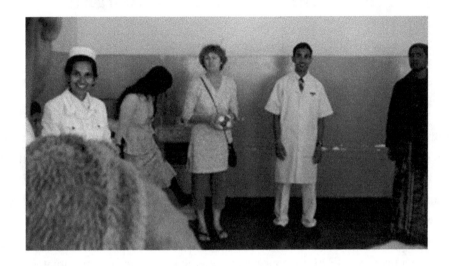

Marjorie teaches the importance of stimulation and activity on the psychiatric ward

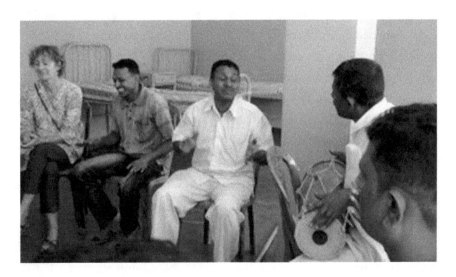

Marjorie and staff bring music and fun to the ward

Chapter 19
New Interactions, New Insights

I delight in the surprise of what is around the corner.

On Saturday nights, Bill and I attended the five o'clock English mass at St Anthony's Catholic Church in the heart of town and following mass, ventured into the market area as dusk gathered. We wandered about the streets bustling full of people shopping before dark fell. Most people living in Nuwara Eliya scampered home to the safety of their families and homes after dark. We did not know if this was customary or a result of the war.

There was one place in town that wasn't empty. At night, Bale Bazaar became a hive of activity for tourists and merchants. Bale Bazaar, situated near a small park in the middle of the town, was a collection of about twenty tiny wooden shops, each about the size of a small bathroom.

Most shops sold the same things: warm coats, winter fleece, mittens and wool hats. Tourists caught unaware by the cold mountain temperatures were willing to pay anything to be warm. One shop sold only pants. A few shops specialised in men's shirts and women's blouses.

The shop merchants all seemed to be outgoing and friendly Muslim men. They all spoke both Tamil and Sinhala, but many merchants spoke some English as well. They demonstrated business acumen and a strong family-style connection amongst themselves.

Rahim was one of these charismatic businessmen. He was about thirty and spoke English. He wanted our rupees, but he made negotiating fun.

"I like this coat, Rahim, but too small. I need bigger size," Bill said in broken English one day as he modelled a coat before a tiny mirror hanging by a string in the shop. Rahim dug into the piles of coats folded into stacks on the floor covered in canvas. Unable to find the right size, he offered Bill a different coloured coat.

"What about this colour?" Rahim asked, holding up a blue coat.

"No, I want red," Bill said.

"What about this one?" asked Rahim, holding up a similar style in a red colour.

"I like this style, but I need bigger," Bill stated, shaking his head.

"I have friend with big size. Wait here." Rahim sped off into the night. He left his shop unattended, and Bill and I continued to paw through the piles of clothing, hoping for the right size. Then, out of the night, Rahim sped back, brandishing a red coat in size L. The other vendors cheered.

Once the item was secured, the bargaining began. Bargaining is part of the culture of Sri Lanka but it is not within the scope of my husband's talents.

"How much?" Bill asked, pirouetting in the mirror with the large red coat.

"Three thousand rupees," said Rahim.

"Oh, I don't know, Rahim. It is thin. Do you think it will keep me warm? I'll give you two thousand rupees."

"Yes, yes, you be warm, but only two thousand rupees? I need to feed my family, Naeae?"

"Twenty-five hundred," Bill countered, shaking his head at the thought of Rahim's starving children.

"Okay," said Rahim like a martyr, but then extending his hand, he grinned. "Very good price, sir. Don't tell anyone." Bill sauntered out of the bazaar wearing his new red coat, his old coat bundled into a bag under his arm. I congratulated Bill on his purchase, and we chuckled at ourselves because we always found ways to justify a warm coat or fleece. We strolled off to supper.

Nuwara Eliya had a good restaurant catering to foreign tourists: the St Andrews Jetwing Hotel. It had a large banquet room, featuring a laden buffet and live music. It was often stuffed with guests from bus tours. Seeking English-speaking company, we did try this venue from time to time, but found it too impersonal.

People on the bus tours had formed friendships already and were uninterested in the quiet Canadian couple sitting alone at their small table. We watched their fun in desolation. Being in a crowd of tourists on holiday served to exacerbate our loneliness and isolation.

Then, we discovered the Coffee Shop in the Grand Hotel. Its moniker was inaccurate. It was neither grand, nor was it a coffee shop. It was a small dining room that served good wine, exquisite food and provided excellent service.

We became regulars on Saturday nights. Their menu featured a curry-crusted dense halibut fillet. Once I tasted it, I never ordered any other entrée. Bill's gastronomy ran towards spaghetti Bolognese and buttered garlic bread.

Other guests in the coffee shop were sparse, but on occasion, we did meet people who were travelling independent of large tours. If we saw a couple, we devised ways to get them to join us.

"Oh, hello, on a holiday?" I'd call over to their table.

"Yes, yes, we are in Sri Lanka for two weeks," said the strange man sitting with his strange wife. "We are from England." The gangly English gentleman turned out to be a lawyer, and his stylish wife was a businesswoman, who sat in a grey woollen coat that had been purchased that evening at Bale Bazaar. Soon, it became awkward to be calling questions and giving responses across the restaurant.

"Listen," I said, gesturing towards our table. "Why don't you join us?"

They seemed happy to have some company and we passed a lovely evening. These encounters happened more than we cared to admit. We sometimes felt needy, hovering around in the Grand Hotel Coffee Shop waiting for unsuspecting tourists who spoke English.

It was desperate, and we knew it. Sometimes, when people declined to join us or when we were the only guests, we came home feeling more dispirited than we did heading out for the evening. However, we were distracted by our upcoming trip to Kandy.

In August, the Kandy Perahera, a nine-day parade, is held in honour of Buddha's sacred tooth. This relic is carried through the streets of Kandy as a processional offering to obtain rain for the cultivation of the crops and for abundance. Kandy is clogged with thousands of tourists for those nine days.

We were really excited to take part in the parade, so we secured accommodation for the Perahera in a guesthouse well ahead in March. Then, we secured a seat for about 5,000 SLRs ($50) through the website of a man named Lal.

We had been instructed to be in our seats five hours before the parade began otherwise proceeding along the streets to our seat would be impossible. As early as nine o'clock, every inch of sidewalk space was crammed with Sri Lankan families sitting on blankets on the concrete, munching their breakfast. We didn't even know free seats existed. These viewers were front and centre.

We had paid for front row seats way back in March. We bought seats for the most expensive *perahera* on the final evening of the parade. We arrived at the pre-arranged time and Lal, the chair seller, promptly placed us in our seats. The plastic deck chairs were placed so close together that the chair arms overlapped.

It was a racket. Promoters tried to sell as many chairs as they could get away with. We started to notice that seating was fluid. As people arrived and bought a seat, they crowded the chairs together even further. They also added additional rows!

Five minutes after we sat down, Lal placed a row of chairs in front of us. "Lal, what are you doing? We paid for front row," I complained.

"Wendy, leave it be," said Bill, trying to pull me back into my plastic chair. He hated confrontation.

"No, we paid for this. This is fraudulent advertising," I said, aggravated by Lal's lack of ethics and Bill's lack of support.

"Ow, Madame." Lal ushered us into the new front row.

"Good, this is even better," I said to Bill. Our chairs were at the edge of the curb.

Then, Lal produced another row of chairs and began setting them up in front of us again. This time he set the chairs up on the road and all the way down the line until he reached the police barricade. The police immediately instructed us to remove the chairs close to the barricade.

As we stood up to drag out seats away, all the other front row seats filled up and, in the end, we had to accept seats placed five rows back. After some more complaining from my part, Lal promised us our money back.

I am not sure if the issue with the chairs spoiled the *rondoli* for me, but it was the longest, most repetitive and most boring parade I have ever seen. It was magnificent for about one hour: whips cracking, dazzling dancers, decorated elephants and drumbeats. For the next four hours, it was whips cracking, dazzling dancers (same dance), decorated elephants and the same drumbeat.

Then, whips cracking, dazzling dancers, decorated elephants and the same drumbeat. Then, again and again. That drumbeat was kind of like the drone of disco. No wonder that people were falling asleep all over the place. Bill and I often caught our chins hitting our chest as well.

After we got back home, I did try and call Lal several times and left his website threatening messages, but he never returned my calls. I felt ripped off. I realised I expected western rules for advanced seating to apply. My ethnocentrism made me feel uncomfortable.

Not much later, I had the chance to gain insight into another Sri Lankan tradition—although, in this case the occasion was not as happy as a parade. Dr Ajith's mother, who was a widow and lived in the family home on a tiny private tea estate about an hour from Nuwara Eliya, was murdered. The police soon arrested a suspect.

One of the women working for Ajith's mother had a boyfriend who was a suspected drug addict. It was believed he had tried to rob her, and she surprised him in an act of thievery. It was shocking.

On the day of the funeral, Chamali and I took a trishaw to the family home to pay our respects. Chamali had instructed me to wear white. Mrs Navaratne was laid out in her bed, dressed in white herself. With grace and dignity, Ajith himself served us tea, giving us a tour of his family home and advising us of the findings of the police.

He was still in deep shock at the brutality and suddenness of his mother's demise. We viewed the body, sipped our cups of tea and left shaking our heads at the horror of a murder. I know these random acts occur in Canada as well, but this was too close to someone I cared about.

After winding down from the tea estate, we stood around the small dusty town awaiting the government bus to come by and haul us back up the hill to Nuwara Eliya. It didn't come. Half an hour later, it still wasn't there. I was squirming in my white shalwar. I had to pee, bad. I looked around for a water closet. I told Chamali my dilemma.

"The bus will come soon, Windy. You must wait," she encouraged.

"I can't," I nearly screamed. I have had five kids. My sphincter wasn't what it used to be, and I had drunk too much tea at the viewing. Darting away from the group, I sped towards a dilapidated concrete structure that stood nearby in a field of weeds and grass.

Alarmed, Chamali hollered, "Windy, come back. You will miss the bus."

Ducking behind the concrete structure, I yanked up my shalwar and wiggling about, I cursed the waistband strings that I'd double knotted that morning to ensure the baggy pants didn't fall off me. Muttering about the incompetence of government that didn't provide adequate facilities for its people, I tore down the pants and squatted in one fluid motion.

Ahh. I watched as the warm, yellow pee sprayed, hitting the weeds I crushed below my feet and my plastic sandals. I cared not. The pee hit the ground so hard it splashed back, splattered my leg in mud. I cared not. I cared not who might have a view.

Drained dry and calm, I tied back the strings at the waist, smoothed down the white funeral shalwar and emerged with dignity from behind the concrete block. Chamali bent her head in shame just as a puff of black smoke heralded the bus cruising into the town.

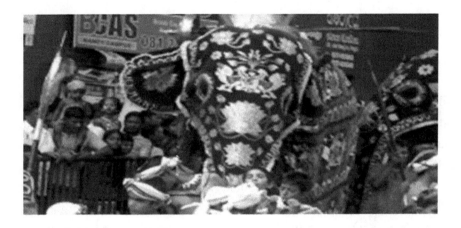

Decorated Elephants for the Kandy Rondoli

Chapter 20
Getting Lost—And Then Finding the Way Out

I love getting lost in a strange city. It is exciting to discover new alleys in the time of being lost and to congratulate myself when I find my way back.

Bill and I didn't always leave Nuwara Eliya on the weekends. We loved hiking and often headed for the emerald green hills around Nuwara Eliya. Mount Pidurutalagala, affectionately referred to as Mt Pedro, soars out of Nuwara Eliya to 8,280 feet of elevation.

It is the highest point on the island of Sri Lanka and can be seen from many parts of the central province of Sri Lanka. Mt Pedro is home base for the central communication systems of the armed forces, the national TV and other important communication devices such as the Civil Aviation Authority. Considered a high security base, it is the site for the main radar unit for the Sri Lanka army.

Daily, as I drove back and forth from work, I noticed this radio tower perched like the king of the castle on the top of the highest peak. I was intrigued. I wondered if there was a trail leading to the tower. I inquired at work and learned that trekking to the top of the hill required a clearance from the Sinhala police. Feeling unable to secure permission based on our limited Sinhala, Bill and I decided to explore the radio tower without permission and without a map.

One Sunday we waved down a trishaw and instructed the driver to take us to the base of the peak. The driver, once he understood our pending plan, began shaking his head and gesturing. Unable to understand his concerns, we shrugged them off. In turn, he also shrugged and drove us to a community on the edge of town.

We hopped out of the trishaw and following the driver's instructions, we wound around a small village alive with pecking hens and small children. We then picked up a steep trail paralleling a rocky creek with wispy, ethereal waterfalls. As we climbed, the trail grew more and more obscure, requiring effort to discern it.

Pushing on, we held thorny branches and vines aside for each other to avoid being lashed in the face. The jungle thickened and the brush grew higher over our heads, like walking through a cornfield.

"I think there are six types of poisonous snakes in Sri Lanka," Bill announced. Unnerved, we dug around in the underbrush and secured a couple of sturdy walking sticks and with each step, whacked the bush alongside to unearth the path and to ward off all the snakes that might show up.

When the path disappeared, we arrested our climb for a reasoned discussion. "Do you think we should continue?" Bill asked, wiping his nose with the back of his hand.

"We are too close now to go back. I think we can create a trail and mark it," I stated with confidence.

Bill bobbed his head, looking about for a way to mark the trail. Something caught his eye. "Hey, what is this?" He stooped, moving aside a giant, decomposing leaf. There, deep in the forest, lurking under a leaf at the top of a steep mountain sat a child's tiny purple sock.

Had someone carried a child up here and had the sock slid from a tiny foot? Did people live up here? It was mysterious. The skin tightened on the back of our necks. We glanced about, and then Bill elegantly slung the purple sock onto a tree branch as a trail marker.

We carried on, banging at the brush as we picked our way along, sometimes a discernible trail, at other times not. Near the top of the hill the jungle thickened, and the brush became almost impossible to penetrate. Our desire was to go on— we were almost there!

However, our confidence was leaking, and our good judgment was whispering that it was time to head back down the hill. We were in an unauthorised military zone. An eerie feeling took over.

Unnerved by the growing darkness, we decided to head back. We spun around. The trail was gone. A frantic search began. Like a tenderfoot, I searched for broken twigs, mashed leaves, or a footprint—anything.

"We just need to go downhill," I reasoned. Slipping and sliding, we pushed and banged our way down through the jungle. Leading the way, the jungle thrashed at Bill's forearms, and he began bleeding as if he'd tormented a cat.

Feeling lost, we rushed and stumbled along. Earlier that day, I had told our landlord's twelve-year-old daughter, Tharushi, that we were attempting the hike. I hoped she understood me and would remember, if we never showed up. I was kicking myself that I hadn't told her father instead.

Suddenly, Bill let out a whoop. A child's purple sock dangled from a branch. Smiling in relief, we embraced in the gloom of the jungle. As we moved back down the hill, the trail materialised with each step and the earlier darkness of the deep jungle lightened as the trees thinned near the base of the hill.

"With risk comes rush," I declared as I patted Bill on the back and swaggered out of the bush onto the road. Bill smiled and shook his head at my folly as he waved down a trishaw to take us home. A risk-taking part of me was manifesting itself in Sri Lanka.

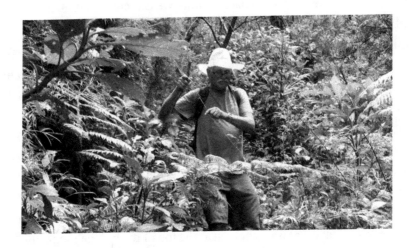

Not lost! Bill hiking down from Mt. Pedro through the lush vegetation

Chapter 21
The Awkwardness Factor—
Avoidance at All Costs

I have a strategy of avoidance. I use it to sit in the shadows and peer out, learning what I need to know and then when I comprehend, I step back out into the limelight.

Living in a foreign country with limited language knowledge, one can't avoid awkward situations, and we had our fair share. When we had negotiated our rent, the price had included utilities. However, our landlord, Sudu Malli, was now concerned about the high consumption of electricity in our little apartment, and without discussing it with us first, he approached VSO for additional funds.

Already at the upper limit of a rent stipend, VSO asked us to make a choice: either pay for the additional costs or move to less expensive lodging. We felt sick about the prospect of a move and knew rental property was difficult to find in Nuwara Eliya. However, in the end we decided that as volunteers, we needed to avoid additional expense and informed VSO of our decision. VSO gave notice to the landlord that we were moving.

A couple of days later, as we entered the yard after some shopping in town, Deelu, the landlord's wife, stepped out from the corner of her home with hands on her hips. She had been waiting for us to come home. She confronted us in the driveway between her home and ours. Her English was not good.

"Why you not like us?" She glared at me. "Why you want move?" She glared at Bill.

"No, Deelu," I assured her. "We like it here. We don't want to move."

Confusion covered her face. "Why you go?"

"We are going because Sudu Malli needs more money for electricity, and VSO cannot pay more money."

Her eyes narrowed. She grabbed me by the arm, shaking her head, "Oh no, no, no, no. You go nowhere. You no pay electricity. You stay."

I had a feeling that the family must have had an awkward conversation that evening. The next day, Sudu Malli approached us, happy and jovial as usual, and requested we not move and told us not to worry about the electrical bills. However, after that, Bill and I were more cognisant of the cost of electricity and only used our little heater at night instead of running it whenever we were home.

Sudu Malli and Deelu made us feel so welcome. We were even invited to their eldest daughter, Tharushi's twelfth birthday party. After we received a tour of their home, decorated in red velour and painted in red, Tharushi insisted I come to her bedroom.

Bill stayed in the basement with Sudu Malli and the other men, including the mayor of Nuwara Eliya. Sudu Malli poured scotch for the boys, and a drumming band played Sinhala songs.

Even though a diminutive eight-year-old, Tharushi was a tour de force. She demanded I play in her room with her. For what felt like hours, we played dolls, ate strange and non-delicious snacks and she showed me all her clothes. I tried to get away, insisting her mother needed help with dinner.

"No, she has a servant. You will stay here because we are going to listen to music now," she commanded. We sat crossed-legged on her bed adorned in frilly pink and listened to music on her pink plastic cassette recorder. "I need to go check on Bill," I advised her after a while.

"No. He is playing with my father and listening to music. We are going to have French fries now." A full forty-five minutes later, her cousin delivered the French fries to her room, and we sat on her bed dipping oven-baked fries into ketchup. I just wanted to be drinking scotch and listening to the music with the men.

Around ten o'clock, Deelu announced dinner was ready. The whirling dervish in her satin crinoline birthday dress escorted me down the stairs. Bill and I, as guests, were served first and sat alone at the huge dining table. While we ate, Deelu stood over us, arms encircling huge bowls of rice and curries.

A few bites into the food and our plates were brimming again. She refused to take no for an answer. I loved the food, and being cursed with a huge appetite, I dug in. Bill, who pecked like a bird at Sri Lankan food, bleated as his plate was filled again and again. He was unable to stem the flow of food from Deelu's curry bowls.

Then, the family and the singers were fed. We smiled and nodded as they ate and conversed in Sinhala and laughed at each other's humour. Often, they looked up to see if we also found it amusing. We smiled and nodded, chuckling gamely, lips straight across, eyes squinting in what we hoped passed for merriment. The awkwardness factor had kicked in hours ago.

"We should go now," I announced.

"No," Tharushi commanded, pointing to an icing-covered slab on the sideboard behind which several large family photos stood framed and propped against the wall. "We haven't had cake yet. You will eat cake."

The food and dishes were cleared away to make space for the cake display. Tharushi danced in anticipation. A massive cake, the size of a coffee table, was unrobed. It was made in Colombo and a cavorting Minnie Mouse had been piped onto it with red, white and black icing.

Tharushi glowed as we sang "Happy Birthday" in English and Sinhala. She blew out every candle with sufficient wind to put out a 3-alarm fire. Proud Sudu Malli waved a knife as he made a small speech we couldn't understand but knew was heartfelt and hospitable.

We smiled and nodded. Then Tharushi presented each person with a piece of cake, but not before, following Sri Lankan birthday tradition, she chomped a bite from each piece.

Licking icing from our lips, I advised Deelu that we needed to go. "She has to open her presents yet," Deelu explained, as she led me to a huge pile of wrapped gifts in the living room. As we sat on the rich red velvet couches with plastic flowers adorning pots in the corners of the rooms, Tharushi removed the bow, then the tape, then the wrapping paper and held the gift high while everyone clapped. She said thank you and proceeded to unwrap the bow from her next gift.

Once the pile of gifts had been reduced to a toy store display, the drumming band struck up in earnest in the living room, their timing affected by the scotch. They sang Sinhala songs, and everyone swayed to the music. Kind Sudu Malli's eyes roamed over Bill and me several times in the evening, checking to see our delight in the party. We smiled and nodded, smiled and nodded.

I sipped fruit punch. Apparently, I was a lady. I can't say I hadn't been warned by that sign about arrack not being sold to ladies which heralded the country attitude around women and drinking. The clock approached 11:30 p.m. Still, my attempts to leave were foiled by both Deelu and Tharushi.

I caught Bill's eye. I cocked my head towards the door. He nodded in secret acknowledgment of the escape plan. We stood in unison and bolted to the door. With one hand on the doorknob, Bill wrestled his way out the door as we hollered our thanks for the delicious meal, wished the birthday girl every success, waved our hands and fled into the night.

It wasn't that I didn't like the family. On the contrary, I loved them very much. They were so kind and thoughtful and hospitable to us. It was just that it was so awkward for us.

We had run away once before for the same reason. A couple of years before we had applied to VSO, Bill and I had decided to learn Spanish. I got the brainy idea that we should sign up for two weeks of Spanish lessons at a language school in Mazatlán.

"In order to really learn the language, we need to do a homestay with a Spanish-speaking family," I said, and Bill half-heartedly agreed. So, we registered for the language school that, in turn, put us in touch with a dentist, Alejandro and his wife, Silvia. We had contracted that they provide us with a room, breakfast and lunch, but we would have our dinner in a restaurant each evening.

Silvia was a vivacious homemaker who took her position seriously. She welcomed us with warm embraces and chattering non-stop in Spanish, she led us through her home decorated in pink draperies and red velvet furniture carved in rich dark wood of vintage Spanish mission design. The formal living room was shrouded in darkness by heavy pink draperies hanging from above nine-foot windows.

She opened our bedroom and pointed out dresser drawers for our clothing. She showed us the brown tiled bathroom where she turned taps, adjusted showerheads and opened cupboards with clean *toallas y bano de papel*.

She beckoned us into the kitchen and flung open the fridge revealing the bowels of the *refridgedora* and advised us of the *manzanas* and other *fruitas y verduras* that sat in the drawers. She turned on the gas range and blasted us with some more unfamiliar words and verbs containing unusual vowels and diphthongs. We could only assume these strange sounds were about the safety features and instructions to operate the gas range.

Once the tour was completed, we retreated to our room and closed the door. We sat on the bed. We stared at each other without saying a word. Bill and I, in preparation for language school, were learning the Spanish alphabet yet did not know a word in Spanish except for 'please'.

Silvia knocked and poked her head into the room. Eyebrows raised, she fired off six questions in a row. Bill and I sat on the bed. We stared at her. Silvia repeated her questions, this time louder. Uncomprehending, we shook our heads. Confused by our lack of response, Silvia closed the bedroom door. We sat on the bed.

Alejandro knocked next and putting his hands on an imaginary steering wheel, drove a car. Understanding he was telling us it was time to go to school, we grabbed our books, waved to Silvia and jumped into Alejandro's car. Alejandro proceeded to give us detailed instructions in Spanish on the best route to school. Along the way, he pointed out his *oficina* and *el restaurante bueno*. We nodded and smiled.

School was thrilling. We nailed the alphabet and learned full words. We learnt to pronounce the Spanish vowels. We met our fellow students, all youngsters compared to us. After school, we went to the beach and then, needing to change for dinner, slid the key in the door at our new home.

Alejandro and Silvia stood on the other side of the door. They waved and smiled and asked questions we didn't understand. We just smiled and nodded and shrugged our shoulders.

The next morning, dawdling in our room, we hatched a plan. We would grab an apple for breakfast, roll a tortilla with *queso* (cheese) for lunch and take off. Unable to find any plastic wrap, we placed the tortilla on a paper towel and rolled it up, stuffing it into our backpacks. We scurried out the door to catch the bus.

Part of the plan consisted of returning home to change into our bathing suits only when we figured Silvia was in *siesta*. After hanging out at the beach, we went for dinner, and we didn't return to our *casa* until we were sure Alejandro and Silvia had retired for the night.

About a week later, during Silvia's presumed siesta time, we eased ourselves into the house. Silvia was standing in the entry with Alejandro, who was home from work early. Alejandro surprised us when he spoke in English.

"We are concerned. You never come home, and you eat nothing. Is everything alright? Have we offended you?" Silvia looked about to cry.

"Oh, no," we protested. "We are just very busy studying," I said in my most scholastic voice.

"We are very happy here," Bill said, smiling. I smiled in support.

"We don't eat much, and we eat out a lot," I said. "We are just very busy," I explained.

"Just busy," Bill agreed, holding up his book bag as evidence.

Silvia brightened after Alejandro translated for her and after that, we made more of an effort to be around. Their granddaughter made her First Communion, and the entire family clan gathered in the house to celebrate. All the extended members of the family spoke to us and asked us questions.

We nodded and smiled. We ate and avoided eye contact. We slunk to our room, just as we did after the birthday party in Sri Lanka. We now realise that by using a strategy of avoidance we moved through these difficult interactions toward a relationship with people that ripened into intimacy.

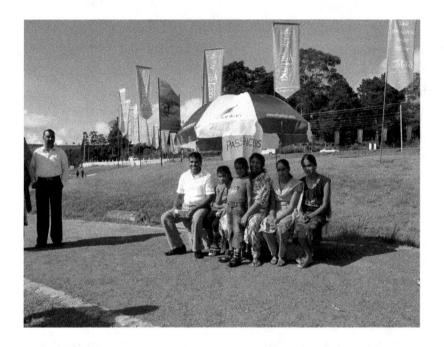

Our landlord's family: Sudu Malli, Deelu, Tharushi, Malisha Perera and their cousins. Sudu Malli passed away a few months after this photo was taken

Chapter 22
On the Move Again

Don't sit too long in one place. You will miss the parade taking place across the street.

As the summer ended, we became restless, and resentment grew. Resentment at the people. At the food. At the markets. At the climate. At Nuwara Eliya. Everything seemed wrong.

At night, we drilled through the stack of DVDs we had brought from Canada at an alarming rate. We retired early because we had no family or friends or extracurricular activities. We were cold but worse still, we were very lonely.

At home, in Canada, we never stayed home. We never watched television. We were always doing something with someone or going somewhere interesting. We had many friends and social activities. It was so different here and so, so bleak.

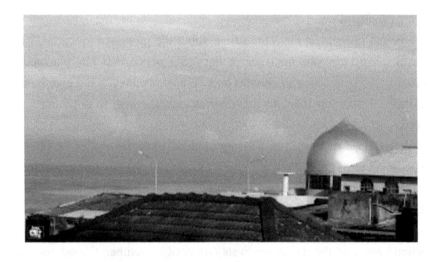

We wallowed in our loneliness. I wanted to go home. So did Bill. By the end of September, our moods were sinking like a stone in a mud puddle.

VSO training had warned us of the inevitability of a point of negativity, a low point. We had been warned that in the process of acculturation, a period or trough would occur when the cultural honeymoon would be over, and negativity and hostility would surface. When we first arrived in Sri Lanka, being stared at was amusing, now we reacted with anger when people stared at us. Initially, we loved the open-air markets and the Sri Lankan food, but now we only saw clutter and jumble in shops and lack of variety on our plates.

"I am sick of the fake hamburgers here," Bill declared one night, shoving his 'hamburger' back onto his plate and chewing with distaste. He always ordered a burger, but it never tasted like home.

I laughed, remembering a passage I'd read from the classic story, *A Passage to India,* by E. M. Forster. In the story, an Englishman living in India was grumbling to himself at a dinner party cooked by Indian servants: "and the menu was: julienne soup full of bottled peas, pseudo-cottage bread, fish full of branching bones, pretending to be plaice, more bottled peas with cutlets, trifle, sardines on toast: the menu of Anglo-India" (p. 45). Here, it was the menu of Anglo-Sri Lanka.

I had my own gripes. "You can't find a damn thing around here," I complained to Bill, when I went searching for a blow dryer in the shops to replace my broken one. We longed for orderly supermarkets and proper stores.

We never believed it would happen to us. But we weren't protected from the trough of acculturation. We had sunk deep, and it felt shitty. We didn't seem to know how to crawl out.

We began pressuring the VSO office about the promised move to Jaffna. I reminded Chandima, our manager in the VSO office that our placement in Nuwara Eliya was to be for six months only. We were now into our eighth month. Technically, I was 'on loan' to this district until the visa to enter Jaffna was obtained.

In August, we renewed our housing contract until the end of October. The VSO plan was to re-apply for a work visa to Jaffna as the government seemed to be becoming more liberal with granting visas for the north. Even the road blockade has been removed—a blockade that had been in place for nearly ten years.

When I was just about to agree to stay on until November, Chandima offered me another possibility of a job in Colombo. Sri Jayewardenepura University in Colombo had been working in partnership with the World Health Organisation

(WHO), the federal government and VSO since 2007 in an attempt to develop a post-baccalaureate diploma program in social work. There were only four trained social workers in the country and yet the Mental Health Policy of Sri Lanka was calling for over two hundred and fifty social workers by 2015.

Due to bureaucratic red tape, the university social work education programs hadn't been able to get off the ground. As I was the only social worker with a PhD in social work in the country, VSO was considering this project as an alternative to Jaffna.

With the help of VSO, I was to help lead a team of doctors, university people and the National Association of Social Workers. We agreed to write curriculum for a certificate program that could ladder people with previous degrees into a Masters of Social Work (MSW). This fast-track method provided the core social work skills. In addition, I was to write a concept paper to deliver to the Senate in hopes of receiving government/ministerial consent for the state university to offer the certificate program as well.

One night, late that fall over dinner at home, we played a game of 'what if'. What if we go to Jaffna? What if we go to Colombo? Bill only made one real contribution to this game. "Anywhere, and the sooner the better," he declared, tugging his red blanket further around his shoulders. I couldn't agree more.

Finally, in October, the Sri Lankan government issued a visa for Bill and me for Jaffna. We were scheduled to leave Nuwara Eliya October 18th. We had a week to pack up our belongings, tie up the dangling loose ends at work and say goodbye.

Before moving north to Jaffna, we had two weeks of Tamil language and cultural training in Colombo. In Jaffna, I was to work in the hospitals and in a clinic called Shanthiham, but VSO also allowed me to continue supporting the post-graduate diploma program. I was pleased to have the opportunity for both tasks.

Despite all my complaining about the weather, I was now feeling a bit nostalgic to leave behind our little house nestled up against the lush green beauty of the Pedro tea estate. I knew I would miss my work and my colleagues. I knew I would miss my Sinhala lessons.

With the short notice to leave Nuwara Eliya, Bill and I plunged into dizzied activity. I focused on getting all ends of my work tied up at the hospital, the community mental health clinic and the community social service agencies. This was the easy part. The hard part was the goodbyes.

I said goodbye to the nurses I had trained in mental health. I got presents. I said goodbye to the community social service workers that I had been training since July. I got presents. I said goodbye to the acute psychiatric staff. I got presents.

I said goodbye to my precious colleagues in the community mental health clinic. I got presents. I said goodbye to the doctors and the psychiatric consultant. I enjoyed my last motorbike ride around Gregory Lake on my last day of work despite the cold, pouring rain that soaked me through.

To say goodbye to Chamali, Bill and I invited her and her husband, Chaminda, to have a meal with us at the Grand Hotel. I savoured my friendship with Chamali along with the last bites I'd ever have of the spicy Caribbean fish dinner. In a moment of emotion and intimacy, I had purchased an amethyst brooch for her.

It was a token of my appreciation of her, her kindness, her collegiality and her goodness to me. A simple brooch couldn't possibly express my love and gratitude.

After we said goodbye to our kind and wonderful landlords, Sudu Malli and his wife Deelu and their children, Tharushi and Malisha, we were done with saying goodbye. It is hard emotional work. I became tearful at times, saying goodbye to people with whom it had been hard work developing a relationship due to differences of language and culture. These people befriended us when we were lonely and cold and sad.

I tried to get all the work done at the hospital: plan and shop for a graduation party, print certificates for over thirty-five graduates in four different programs, correctly spell the long names, hand over the budgets I had been responsible for, complete the closing report, provide hard and soft copies of my lectures for Chamali, and have documents translated into Sinhala.

In the meantime, Bill was packing up the house with uncharacteristic enthusiasm and speed. His industry at this task resulted in some concern. Three days before we were to leave, there was not a dish left unpacked, which made eating difficult. Two days before we left, we slept on blankets spread out on the bed as all bed sheets had been whisked into cardboard boxes.

Boxes were stacked everywhere, and dirt was abundant. He swept under the bed, bookshelves and sofas. Piles of flies and dust were evidence of his efforts.

I was so grateful for all his preparation. Come moving day, we had time for one last walk in the lush green tea estates. We walked hand in hand, saying goodbye to our life and our home for the past ten months. Then, heading back to our little white home for the last time, I scrubbed down the kitchen and mopped the floors while Bill loaded the van waiting to take us to Colombo.

Goodbye, cold and wet Nuwara Eliya! Goodbye, kind and good people! In both Sinhala and the Tamil language, there is an expression used to say goodbye. In these languages, people do not say goodbye; the saying is more of an invitation.

The expression in Sinhala is *gihin ennan*, and in Tamil it is *poittu vaareen* and both mean something like 'Go and come again'. We were about to go, and we hoped we could come again.

In Colombo at the VSO office, we met three new members of the VSO team. Anne Murray, a business consultant from Scotland, Dr Marcia Brophy, a child psychologist from the UK and Mary Cuttle, another business consultant from Scotland. Jo Coombs, an occupational therapist and Mark Chamberlain, both from England, were scheduled to arrive soon.

After the introductions and securing a schedule, the van driver drove us to a small two-bedroom apartment called Asian Court in Colombo 04, a desirable Colombo address, close to Galle Face Green and Cinnamon Gardens. The apartment was previously used by a VSO volunteer who had since returned to his home country. VSO had decided to keep it as a 'guest house' for VSO volunteers visiting Colombo for meetings and trainings.

It was not the most ideal place, as it was some distance to the VSO office, but we only had to tolerate it for a couple of weeks. Its saving grace was a tiny view of the ocean. If we stepped out onto the small patio, we looked over the rounded golden dome of a mosque to the wavy blue Indian Ocean beyond.

We commenced our language training, this time in Tamil. Sinhala and Tamil are different languages, with a different alphabet and a different sound. Sinhala is sing-songy while Tamil is more staccato.

I felt bad to leave Sinhala behind as I had worked hard to learn the little I did know. I thought that I could find a new Sinhala teacher in Jaffna, but soon realised the impossibility of learning both languages at the same time.

In November, having completed our training, Mary, Marcia, Bill and I packed up and made our way to Jaffna. We rented a van and set out from the thronging noise and bustle of Colombo, back through three important cities known as the Cultural Triangle. As we travelled further north, we swapped the knowledge we had gleaned from our induction training and additional readings to better understand the situation in the north.

It was sobering to go through Elephant Pass, the military division line that kept the north separated from the south of the country for so many years. We were nervous. Mystery shrouded Jaffna due to its long isolation from the world.

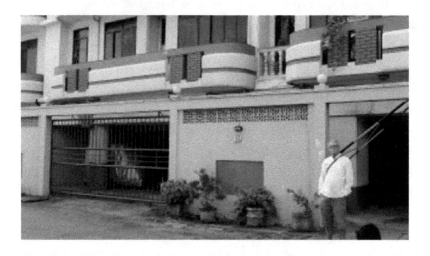

Asian Court: Our temporary apartment in Colombo where we stayed during our in-country preparation to go to Jaffna. The view of the Indian Ocean was lovely

Part Three
Living North of Elephant Pass

Chapter 23
New Climate, New Home, New Friends

Ah, sunshine. It drives lizards to sit on rocks, cats onto windowsills and humans to turn their faces upward.

Arriving in Jaffna, we settled into Thinakkural Rest, a guesthouse on Chetty Lane, until we found permanent accommodation. We unpacked a few clothes and work materials, but most of our belongings remained in cardboard boxes stored in our tiny room. After stowing our belongings, we took a little walk before nightfall.

Jaffna was what we expected, and yet, not what we expected. The humidity was so high we walked about drenched in sweat. However, the combination of humidity and heat produced lush tropical palmyra palms, colourful flowers and warm soothing breezes.

Grace and beauty imbued the architecture. Homes were spacious, genteel, rancher styles with large verandas and sizable, gated yards. Several times a day, large loudspeakers mounted outside the mosques that dotted the peninsula blared chants of prayer into the steamy air.

Despite the beauty, racial tensions as well as fear and distrust of government permeated Jaffna. The stony-faced Sri Lankan Army stood on every street corner, uniformed and hefting heavy rifles. It was shocking to see the shelled and abandoned homes that lay in ruins from the war. Voracious tropical plants had taken over, the vines covering fences and concrete walls and snaking through broken windowpanes.

Displaced people were forced to remain in refugee camps. People had lost limbs and were disfigured from bombings and shelling. People had been tortured. Many had family members who had 'disappeared'.

In 1999, a United Nations study stated that Sri Lanka had the second highest number of disappearances in the world. The 'disappeared' are those believed to be forcibly detained by armed men or the army during the civil conflict. By 2003, the Red Cross reported receiving twenty thousand complaints of disappearances in Sri Lanka.

In 2016, the Sri Lankan government issued sixty-five thousand Certificates of Absence, thus allowing family to manage property and the assets of those who had disappeared. Despite Sri Lanka's Office of Missing Persons, families have received few answers about the whereabouts or demise of their loved ones, and they feel betrayed by the government.

With this collective trauma, the way things were in the old Jaffna was gone. The intelligentsia had fled, and the people still living there were traumatised. As a Tamil man we had met in Canada put it, "This is not Jaffna anymore. Jaffna is in Canada, Australia and Singapore." I wondered what was ahead of me.

As we strolled around, everything seemed so unfamiliar. I wasn't prepared for the striking differences between the north and south within such a tiny country.

I knew that we were heading into a war-torn area of the country. I knew the people were racially Tamil and spoke the Tamil language. I knew that this area had been closed off to the rest of the world for nearly thirty years, but I knew these things at an intellectual level, rather than at an emotional level.

I had worked hard to learn Sinhala and to read the Sinhala alphabet and expected this to help me navigate in this new town. However, there were no Sinhala signs. All signage was in Tamil. Despite being a tri-lingual country, little English was evident here.

I couldn't order a trishaw anymore, I couldn't read a menu, and I couldn't find my way about the town; it was a maze of walled houses and streets and tiny shop after tiny shop.

The people seemed different too. I had grown accustomed to the Sinhala race and culture. Tamil people seemed more abrupt, and yet more boisterous in their speech, actions and emotions. They were less infatuated with white folk and passed by us without looking at us or making a fuss.

They appeared to be more animated with each other and seemed to enjoy life more. As a race, their skin is generally darker in colour, whereas Sinhala people are more of a range of colour from quite fair to very dark. Clothing styles were similar in both regions, although in Jaffna, unmarried women and young girls wore the *shalwar kameez*.

I didn't realise the food was going to be so different as well. Sinhala food is downright bland compared to the Tamil cuisine. It is not only the spicing that is different, but the type of foods too: *dosais, pittu* and more seafood.

As we experienced our new home, we marvelled at the cars, the landscape and the town. Morris Minor cars came to the tiny island in the 1930s and still motored about town. The isthmus landscape was so very different from anything I had ever seen. I didn't anticipate the bird sanctuaries stretching for misty miles and providing a home for the Ibis and Painted Stork, among hundreds of other shore birds. Despite Jaffna's population of over six hundred thousand people, the downtown itself suggested nothing more than a large village.

The next morning, over a breakfast of eggs and curry, we discussed our assignments. Marcia and I were mental health professionals, and we had been assigned to work for a partner organisation called Shanthiham. Mary, who worked for the governance arm of VSO, would be assisting to develop shelters and empower women exposed to family violence.

Marcia and I walked the few blocks to Shanthiham. A large gate and fencing protected the property. Inside the gate, the yard boasted lush palms and verdant gardens, its plants and flowers swaying in the tropical breeze. A palapa gazebo with a sand floor sat to the left of the building. A dozen chairs were placed in a circle within the palapa.

The office was a two-story home, converted into offices. We entered the building and introduced ourselves. A middle-aged woman in a blue sari moved from behind the desk to greet us, "Vanukuum, Doctor Brophy and Doctor Nordick." She bowed, her intelligent eyes taking in the new staff. "I am Sivarani," she said with fluent English.

"Vanukuum," we replied, bowing in kind.

Gracefully, she ushered us up a wide flight of stairs to the office of the Executive Director. "Here is the ED's office," she indicated with her hand. She rapped on the door, and a small, thin man opened it.

"I'm the ED here," he said, offering us his hand. His real name was never disclosed.

The ED had been working on some accommodation options for us, so that afternoon, we set out to look at apartments. Marcia, Bill and I did not want to live together, so we needed to find two separate places. In the end, we found a large two-story home with kitchens on both floors, which the landlord agreed to make into two separate apartments by sealing the inside staircase between the floors and installing an outside staircase to make a separate entrance.

It took about two weeks for the renovations on the apartments to be completed, so Thinkurral Rest became home for a little while longer. That first week, Bill, Marcia, Mary and I tried out a little pub on Temple Road, which was listed in the Lonely Planet as a hangout for expats. We figured we might get to know the lay of the land by meeting other people working for NGOs in the area.

That night, over drinks in the covered outdoor patio, we met a tiny, Japanese woman named Mitsuko. She spoke very good English and told us she was working for a Japanese NGO called Parcic. Parcic provided livelihood restoration to fishermen who had lost their boats and fishing gear during the Asian tsunami that hit the northern coast of Sri Lanka on Boxing Day 2004.

Mitsuko shared a home with Gerd, an Albanian who had immigrated to Germany. Gerd was working for the UN Food Program and was situated in Jaffna due to the war. Mitsuko offered an invitation, "Gerd and I have a yoga teacher come to our home Monday through Thursday mornings at six o'clock. Would you like to join us?" she asked.

"We will be there," we all agreed.

The next morning, we arrived at Gerd and Mitsuko's home. It was a large, one-story home with a beautiful veranda encircling the front and side. A security guard greeted us at the rickety gate, and we wheeled our bicycles into the yard. We propped the bikes against a tree that stood in the garden.

There we met the handsome Gerd, who was preparing coffee for us, and our Tamil yoga teacher, Shiva. Shiva practiced an interesting type of yoga that involved strange breathing practices.

"Breathe in deeply from your belly to your head. Hold your breath until you can feel the millions of termites crawling around in your head," he instructed. "Pant like a dog, sucking through your teeth," he chanted. We then did a sequence of rapid movements that involved imagining ourselves as 'little green worms'. He also advocated a lot of swinging and twisting of our bodies.

Marcia, a devoted yoga practitioner told us later, "I've done a lot of yoga, but I've never had anyone teach flinging like that and call it yoga."

Gerd had convinced Shiva to teach us Tamil following our yoga lesson. Shiva was a kind man and although not a teacher of language, he devoted himself to the task. He drew the Tamil alphabet on a white board on the front porch as we sipped the Italian coffee Gerd served us each morning. Slowly, the 'green worms' grew stronger and they learned phrases and words in Tamil.

Bill joined us for the yoga but jammed again on the language training. Soon, Mitsuko approached him to teach English to her colleagues at Parcic. Within a week, he had a slew of students lining up to learn English and not just from Parcic.

The students were at different levels of English, so, free of charge, he offered two beginner and two intermediate English lessons a week. He worked hard to create material and a learning approach that suited his students. Technically not cleared by the government to work or volunteer, he joked he was "just having coffee with a group of new friends."

I was proud of him. He recognised the importance of his students learning English to improve their employment opportunities. He took his teaching responsibilities seriously.

One weekend, Bill and I decided to cycle over to Gerd's house, with the intent of inviting him out for a bike ride. Gerd shook his head, "I don't have a bicycle or a scooter." Then, he had an idea. "My guard has a bike. I'll see if I can borrow it," he said, dashing towards the guardhouse.

He emerged with a crooked grin, pushing a rusty Lumala bike. We all headed down Temple Road after the security guard closed the gate behind us. We cycled out towards the north of Jaffna to the sea.

We crossed a long bridge that linked the mainland to an island, and as we crested the top of the bridge, we began sailing down the rutted hill. Gerd's bike had no brakes. Gerd lifted his feet off the pedals, stuck out his legs to the sides, hung on to the handlebars, and careened down the hill avoiding the ruts coming at him at high speed. His dark hair tousled in the wind, and he shouted in sheer exhilaration. "Ahhhhhhhhhhh." We laughed at his folly. We had made a friend.

On 15 November, our Yaalpaanum (Tamil for Jaffna) house was ready for occupancy. The shelled house had been renovated into two suites. The upper floor was for Marcia and the downstairs was for Bill and me.

Our new home had a large yard, its own water well, an outdoor squat toilet and a hearth in the kitchen for cooking. Bill and I had three large bedrooms and a regular toilet inside!

Our furniture and motor scooter arrived, and we moved into the house on a Tuesday morning. With the renovations completed, a sense of settling arose. We knew where to find an item, and we no longer needed to dig it out of a musty cardboard carton.

Our VSO furniture, a garbage can, a couple of tables and a desk provided a new sense of organisation. Bill strung his laundry lines and puttered about repairing our bicycles and hanging pictures as directed.

After his months of freezing in Nuwara Eliya, Bill basked outdoors. He sat reading in a plastic lawn chair beside a newly purchased plastic patio table. Playful squirrels, red-headed woodpeckers pecking at the jackfruit tree, and lizards stretched out along tree branches made up his garden friends.

A mongoose visited, eating the vegetable peelings I threw into a compost pit. Inside the home, we had our own giant pet gecko, Gary.

Gary lived in a wooden beam that ran across the ceiling between our entry and our living room. Gary would emerge from a small hole in the beam like clockwork every evening once the sun was down. One night, we saw him on his beam.

He was motionless, mesmerised, watching a white moth fluttering around the uncovered light bulb on the ceiling. Then he opened his mouth, and in a flash, a long fuzzy tongue unfurled, slurping up the moth. We both gasped. Gary hadn't moved but was smacking his lips, a small corner of moth wing dangling as he chewed. We expected a belch of satiation. Gary seemed to like us, and we liked him. If he stayed on his beam, I figured he was good entertainment.

As we were the new tenants, other critters had to be moved out. Bill was my exterminator. He had developed a rapid response to my cry of 'Bug Patrol'. The Bug Patrol was constantly removing five-inch centipedes, one-inch caterpillars, baby frogs, grasshoppers and other assorted and sundry buggy-type critters coming into the house for a visit. The removal was all done with hands encased in toilet paper.

Sri Lankan cities are riddled with cockroaches. Strolling home after dinner, cockroaches noisily scuttled beneath our feet. They didn't just stay on the streets. They rattled into our apartment under doorways and through open windows. Bill was the cockroach killer.

He would give the hideous bugs a substantial shot of Mortein spray, a white poison, whilst shouting, "Bastards." Within seconds, the beetles would roll over onto their back, legs wiggling up in the air and then, expire in seconds. Then Bill, fingers encased in white toilet paper, would pick up the expired creatures and drop them into the toilet with a triumphant flush.

At five o'clock, like clockwork, the mosquitos droned through the windows to feast on our blood. We were still lucky compared to our friend Kamal, who had had a nest of dengue mosquitos roosting in the humidity of her bathroom. And she had had the misfortune of being harassed by many other creatures.

"Bloody Hell," she exclaimed each time she told a story of a new creature in her house. A cobra had slithered into her kitchen. She moved. She had a hoard of wild boars in her garden. She moved. She had to keep moving to keep safe from the wildlife. I decided I could live with a couple of centipedes, frogs and cockroaches.

Each day, thousands of bats dangled in St John's Old Park like drab globes on a dead Christmas tree. At first, I thought they were crows. However, as dusk gathered, these nocturnal 'crows' would begin responding to an ancient and instinctive calling. As they fluttered and stirred, the shape of their wing startled me.

It was scalloped. I saw the brown of the breast. I smelled the smell. I heard their sonar sounds from a distance as they took wing in search of mosquitoes, flies and fruit. At first glance, they resembled a flock of Canadian geese flying south in preparation for winter.

They were fascinating to watch. In the evening, they swooped into our garden. We were glad we had had our rabies shots before leaving Canada.

The house began to feel like home. Each morning, Bill played loud rock music or danced in the sunlight singing an off-key version of Bob Marley's *Buffalo Soldier*. Opening the blinds allowed morning sunlight to flood in. No longer were we struggling to keep warm.

Bill had abandoned his blanket for shorts and T-shirt. This was the tropical climate we had imagined when starting our CUSO adventure.

Even though I had never been a sweaty person, in the heat of the Jaffna sun and under the weight of oppressive humidity, every pore in my body leaked. Moisture streamed down my legs, pooling in my sandals. Water leaked from around my waistline, leaving my shirt and waistband soaked.

I had always eschewed patterned clothing, but I now sought out patterned tops as they disguised dark sweat stains. For the first time in my life, I was wishing I had more of a moustache to soak up the dew on my upper lip. My neck was slick, and my hair damp and limp. Just like Sri Lankan people, I began carrying a dew rag.

Three wobbly, noisy house fans spun all day and night with little cooling effect. After work, I cycled home, showered (again) and changed into the closest thing to naked: a baggy, patterned muumuu frock. Bill too, struggled with the heat.

At night, we lay prostrate under the mosquito net, looking at the banana palm hanging limply outside the window begging for a breeze. We languished like old dogs. We had moved from the Arctic to the Sahara Desert.

In January, monsoon season arrived. The day-long, bone-rattling rain of mountainous Nuwara Eliya was different from the Jaffna rains. In Jaffna, the skies opened and sheets of water dumped from the clouds like God pouring from an ocean-sized bucket. One day, I hopped on my bicycle leaving work in search of lunch and was caught in a downpour.

Despite diving under a huge leafy tree that I shared with another cyclist, I was drenched. The downpour lasted a good ten minutes and then, as suddenly as is began, the rain stopped. The sun poked out, the clouds dissipated, and the sun's glint left trees shimmering.

Birds shrieked in the trees. The heat began to build again. The streets ran deep with water. With little choice, I cycled home through deep muddy brown puddles for a change of dry clothes. I didn't mind. The rain was warm and so was the day.

As we all adjusted to the climate, our little band of expats became good friends. Bill and I hosted a dinner party. Lal, the little VSO cook from Colombo, had given me a photocopied booklet of his favourite recipes. That night, I slaved over the recipes contained in the booklet.

Soft rock, played from a disc on my computer, filtered out of the barred windows into the garden. In the warmth of the evening, the palms swayed and night birds cooed. We sipped wine and ate dinner on the patio. The warmth of the air was as warm as the relationships that were forming.

The only time we felt lonely was around Christmas. Christmas represents so much to me: the mystery of the Divine Messiah, the magic of Santa Claus, and the beauty of decorated trees and the glow of coloured lights. Christmas is the joy of family time and the fun of friends. It is the hustle and bustle, the anticipation, the wonder of a snowfall and the awe of Christmas Eve. It is the sentiment in the carols and the gift of traditions.

Just before moving to Jaffna, Bill and I had visited the Cinnamon Grand Hotel in Colombo. We were just crossing the marbled grand lobby of the hotel, when we caught sight of all the Christmas trees, decorated for the holidays. The lobby was filled with the tunes of *I'll Be Home for Christmas.* Out of nowhere, I was weeping.

The trigger of the white Christmas trees festooned with orange and blue balls tore at the defence mechanisms I had put in place. I knew I wouldn't be decorating a tree and I wouldn't be with my family and friends for Christmas.

Luckily, Gerd hosted a Christmas party. His wife, Maria, had returned from Germany with their son, and she had decorated their home in Christmas tradition. As we sipped wine on the patio, some Christmas carollers strolled down Temple Road, dressed like Santa but who looked more like Krampus. We hollered at them to sing to us and before we knew it, ten masked Krampuses flowed into the yard, dancing on the deck to *Jingle Bells*.

On Christmas Day, I phoned my sister, Teresa, moaning about not being home for Christmas. Teresa chided me, "You don't hold the monopoly on crying at Christmas, Wendy, just because you are in Sri Lanka. For many years, I didn't get to come home for Christmas as the roads were too dangerous with snow or my kids were too small or I had to work."

Then, in empathy, she confided, "I only have to put on Christmas carols and do some Christmas baking and I am 'whaaing' all about the house. We Nordicks, are all the same, when it comes to Christmas," she said. It was true. I decided to play some carols and decorate our banister and our tree. Even though it eased our homesickness a bit, we were glad when Christmas was over.

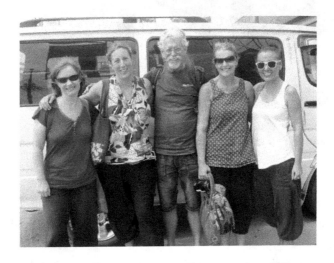

Jaffna Family L to R: Mary Cuttle, Jo Coombs, Bill, me and Dr. Marcia Brophy

Chapter 24
Learning and Researching

The more I know, the more I learn, the more I realize I don't know.

Marcia and I had only just begun working for Shanthiham, and as part of our orientation, we were invited to attend a training session entitled 'Mental Health and Psychosocial Support in Conflict and Post Conflict', sponsored by the Peace Building and Development Institute of Sri Lanka. They offered local and international initiatives in capacity building and research for areas where armed conflict has impacted the people.

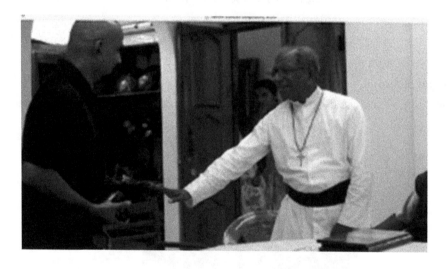

Father Damian and trainer from Peacebuilding and Development Institute of Sri Lanka

This course clarified for me what was needed in the region. It was also an opportunity to network with those already providing psychosocial care in the community.

As part of this training, we attended three locations: a church, an orphanage and a beach. At the church, we met a Catholic priest, Father Damian, who provided support and helped organise post-traumatic therapy for those affected by the war. He helped 'his people' advocate for government funding and jobs and garnered support for people to return to livelihoods such as fishing that were destroyed by the war.

The day we visited the church, he asked some of his clients to speak about their experiences during the war. Some stood and told us how they had to flee when the Indian Army besieged Jaffna. Others, more shy or reluctant, spoke no more than a few words, yet even in their poverty of speech they conveyed terrible images. "Mother was shot before my eyes" or "I saw dogs eating the bodies."

My heart slammed into my chest, and I couldn't breathe. Tears slid down my face. A tiny woman, no larger than a child, stood to speak. Her sari was draped about her body, amplifying her thin stature. She began to speak in Tamil, and Father Damian translated for us.

"My whole family was shot by the Indian Army, even my baby..." Shockingly, she began to seizure, her body trembling as she fell to the ground slumping into unconsciousness. The flashbacks and memories had overwhelmed her.

It wasn't hard to recognise the severe level of trauma. Marcia and I exchanged grimaces, and I could see that she felt as overwhelmed as I did. *What are we doing here?* we asked ourselves.

The woman's friends lifted her slight body and moved her into another room to recover. Father Damian explained that she was traumatised but she had really wanted to tell us her story. Clearly, she was a long way from being able to do so. Father Damian continued his orientation and explained how priests had fed and hid Tamil people in village churches from the Indian and Sri Lankan Army.

Father Damian stroked the small wooden crucifix that hung from his neck and shook his head as he explained the plight of war widows. "Women without husbands are forced to form relationships with the Sinhala soldiers who patrol the areas. They exchange sex for rice and food to feed themselves and their families."

"Sometimes these relationships are business arrangements while others are 'love relationships', but cultural pressures make it difficult to legitimise these relationships. The women remain beholden to the men that exploit and support them at the same time. The larger community shuns the women for the alliance and refuses to assist them." Single women were caught between a rock and a hard place.

Children's education was also affected by the poverty of the area. Parents were often unable to afford compliance with government regulations requiring school uniforms. In addition, the cost of transportation and the distance to a school created barriers to education.

The second field location was a Hindu temple, where an orphanage had been set up. Close to forty children ranging in age from five to seventeen performed a song for us in the courtyard. It was beautiful and well-rehearsed.

The director of the orphanage, a Hindu priest, explained that many of the children had lost their parents during the war or their parents were unable to care for them out of poverty. Their beautiful brown eyes seemed to reflect sorrow. I found I could not make eye contact, as I couldn't bear their pain and loss.

Finally, we were taken to Point Pedro beach. The wind blew off the ocean and whipped our hair and flapped the coloured *pallu*s of the Tamil women's saris. We stood in the white sand looking out at the muddy Indian Ocean.

Our tour director pointed across the water. "Tamil Nadu in India is just 19 kilometres across the water. There are sixty million Tamil people living there."

The Sri Lankan government was fearful of the massive potential of these Indian Tamils providing support to the Tamil Tigers, so the Sri Lankan Army guarded the beach all around Jaffna. The buildings on the beach stood shelled or in complete disrepair. The families were forced inland.

Raj, our facilitator for the tour, pointed to his feet, bent down and fished something cylindrical from the sand. He held up an unexploded bullet.

"Watch your step," he cautioned, with a smile.

All eyes turned down, peering into the sand. Spent bullet shells lay everywhere on the sand. A battle had taken place here, on this beautiful beach. He then explained that most of the unexploded shells were rendered useless by the corrosion of the salt water in the waves that crashed along the beach.

As we climbed back into the van, I reflected on what I had seen that day. Who was I to even begin to believe that I could assist in the face of so many traumas? I chastised myself. What can I offer people who had lost family, limbs, land and remained oppressed by their government?

I hoped that the principles of therapy were somewhat universal. I prayed the adage to be true: "God doesn't call the prepared, he prepares the called." *Prepare me, Lord*, I muttered in silent prayer in my tiny chapel throughout the coming days.

After the training, I had a greater picture and context of the enormous collective trauma of the region of Jaffna. I settled into my office. Bright green palms tapping against the window belied the horrors of the past years of war.

My desk consisted of a table covered with a plastic tablecloth and a mammoth chair that didn't allow my legs to slide under the table. Here, I began developing an outline of my assessment plan.

The plan first involved research to identify the needs and the strengths in the community. First, I consulted with my colleagues to determine what organisations and community services already existed and started to make a list. Then I contacted as many of the people or organisations as possible and interviewed them.

The interview would focus on their mandate, the types of services they provided, and the gaps in service. I also outlined my skills and education and asked how I might be of service to the community. Finally, I planned an analysis of the gathered information and used it to develop a plan of action.

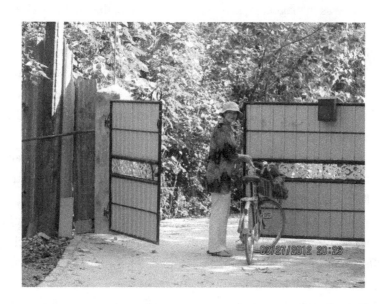

2012: Leaving for work at Shanthiham on my bicycle through our garden gate in Jaffna

I wasn't at my desk much for the next few weeks, as I scootered about the Jaffna Peninsula doing my research and taking extensive notes. I interviewed key personnel working in the field. I visited the acute care hospital in Tellipalai, a suburb of Jaffna.

I spoke with staff at a mental health group home and a government social worker who bridged the gap between the community and the hospital. I spoke with community care workers and other local NGOs supporting vocational retraining, housing projects, women's groups, widows and disability organisations. I spoke with health officers and community counsellors.

Shanthiham had been responding to the needs of the war-affected in Jaffna since 1987. However, the 'trauma team' at Shanthiham were mostly para-professionals or held degrees in disciplines other than social work or counselling. Over the thirty years of war, international NGO support had been offered to Shanthiham staff.

They had received training in assessment, psychosocial first-aid, counselling and other related skills, but they told me that most of the training had been delivered in short blocks of time, such as a weekend. No systematic building of theory or skills had taken place over time. With my previous experience assessing the community in Nuwara Eliya, I now recognised the need to focus on a plan that was manageable, achievable and sustainable in the twelve months I had remaining in Sri Lanka.

The therapeutic dynamic was that the people of Jaffna needed to learn to cope, find hope, recognise their strengths and resilience, heal, adjust and move forward after the devastation of war. Psychosocial support, mental health and counselling were my expertise, but I couldn't be everybody's therapist. I realised my primary role was that of training the trauma team staff.

Teaching them would empower them, empower the community and most critical of all, would leave the skills operational in Jaffna after I returned to Canada. This was sustainable development.

I concluded that zigzagging between the field (where they applied the knowledge) and the classroom (where they received supervision, coaching and new skills) was the best approach for training. This support seemed the most effective route and a standard of best practice. The previous format did not allow for the shaping and mentoring or reflexive practice that can develop a counsellor into an effective therapist.

I submitted my project proposal to VSO and was given a green light to proceed, accompanied by a yellow card of caution that my plan was, perhaps, 'too ambitious'. The biggest hurdle I saw was how to train Tamil-speaking people. Some of the staff had limited English, but I needed to teach conceptual theory and practice skills that required a higher vocabulary.

Luckily, I remembered that I had, in fact, already met someone who could help me. Some months earlier, Bill and I had attended a party at the British Embassy in Kandy. At that party, I had met a lawyer, Mick, who was soon moving to Jaffna. He had told me his wife, Vasuki, was a Sri Lankan Tamil.

Now all I had to do was send Mick an email asking him if his wife might be open to teaching me Tamil. The next day, Mick called and advised his wife was willing to teach.

In her home, Vasuki set up a classroom. She was bright, sunny and organised. She was a speech pathologist and used her speech pathology knowledge to assist us with enunciation. Knowing where the tongue needed to be placed in the mouth was important to make correct Tamil sounds. I loved her teaching method and made progress.

Vasuki also agreed to translate for me three times a week. However, as yet, I had no budget to pay her. After some research on NGOs with a mandate to support trauma-based organisations in Sri Lanka, I developed a budget proposal and submitted it to USAID, an organisation that had provided trauma therapy training to Shanthiham in the past.

Within a few weeks, USAID approved the funding, so I could hire a translator—Vasuki. Shanthiham wrote up the contract and administered the funds. Vasuki and I became a seamless, enthusiastic team: I taught in English, and she translated in Tamil. I felt I now had the infrastructure in place to proceed and felt less alone with Vasuki in the classroom.

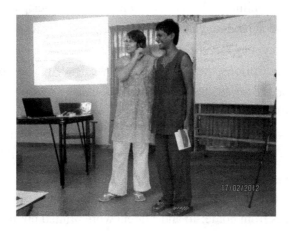

Vasuki Rajasingham translating for me as I taught the mental health course and therapy skills

Chapter 25
Feeling Vulnerable

Blustering our way through life is a false economy. We are living a lie. By hiding our fragility and our vulnerability we rob ourselves of receiving the divine support only available through others.

In January, Jo Coombs joined the VSO team in Jaffna. Jo was an occupational therapist from the United Kingdom and was assigned to work on the psychiatric ward at the Tellipalai hospital near Point Pedro. Once Jo arrived and settled into the 'Jaffna family', as we called ourselves, we began planning excursions. We each had a VSO scooter and on Sundays or Poya days (the full moon days, which are public holidays), we often ventured out onto the islands.

We had all heard from colleagues about Chetty Beach, (Charty Beach to the locals), a spot out on the islands that was a good place to swim. It is at the edge of an isthmus, facing the Indian Ocean. The road to Chetty Beach veers off the main road that links all the islands together and then heads left over a rutted road towards a deserted military checkpoint. Our trishaw driver parked in the sand near the beach and agreed to wait while we swam and picnicked.

About a dozen young men from the Sri Lanka Navy were wading in the water in their underwear. Curious, they watched us as we headed to the concrete change rooms situated on the beach. The newer-looking change rooms were locked, and the door hung off the toilet facilities.

The toilets were squats filled with faeces hardened in mounds. There were no water buckets to rinse the toilets. It seemed that scraps of clothing wadded up in the corner had been used for tissue by previous bathers.

Disgusted, we used the concrete walls for privacy screens to change. We all wore bathing suits from home: Jo and Marcia wore printed bikinis, Mary wore a one-piece bathing costume, and I wore a tankini. Bill wore long swim trunks.

The local men gathered near the shore and moved to the side as we tested the water. The water was dark and muddy-looking, but the temperature lured us like a warm bath. It was wonderful. Sighing and allowing our stress to dissipate, we floated, our bodies buoyant in the salty water. We chattered to each other, trying our best to ignore the young men who crept in ever closer.

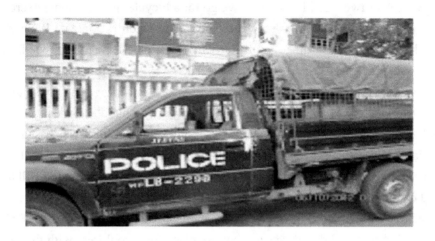

Jaffna Police Department where I made my sexual assault report

As we floated about, we looked further down the beach to see Sri Lankan women wading in the water, their long, wet saris clinging to their legs. The beach there was full of litter and seaweed. It became clear to us then that the men and women didn't swim together.

Bill engaged in conversation with the young men wading nearby as best he could, but some of them were disrespectful and swam too close to us, often trying to cop a feel under the water. We had to be quite stern with them to leave us alone.

"Go away," Marcia said. Smiling, the men backed away a bit, but didn't leave us alone. One man, emboldened to score, reached towards Marcia's body. "Fuck off," tiny Marcia screamed at him. Some words seem international. The men turned away and started showing off their muscular strength by tossing each other about and making human pyramids from which to dive.

Later, as I lay in the sun on my beach towel, I realised how much it bothered me that the Sri Lankan women were assigned to the crummy, weedy beach. It bothered me that they didn't have functional bathing attire. Swimming fully dressed seemed a way to avoid judgment or repercussions from perceptions that the woman had enticed a man toward her.

It seemed it was the woman's responsibility to keep herself safe, rather than the men's responsibility to be appropriate. Women continue to be blamed for the consequences of gender and systemic inequality.

A week or two later, I suggested we go for a bicycle ride, get some exercise and explore our surroundings. However, the weather didn't cooperate. Monsoon rains had poured all morning. Finally, around two o'clock, the rain stopped. Bill and I swung by Gerd's place on Temple Road.

Clad in rain gear, we headed off out onto the causeway that links Jaffna proper to a series of islands. We cycled through deep puddles, splashed mud, tried to avoid water-filled ruts, dodged buses and waved at folks we passed.

Early into our bumpy ride, and for the third time since arriving in Jaffna, I punctured my rear tire. Not wanting to spoil everyone's fun, I insisted Bill and Gerd continue with their explorations while I walked my bike back to town. We agreed to meet later at an ice-cream parlour called Rio Ice-cream on Point Pedro Road. We had heard that it was a favourite place for a cool treat with the local and expat crowd.

On the causeway leading back to Jaffna, I passed an army/navy bunker that had been erected during the war. An armed guard in a blue shirt and pants was posted in front of the guard shack. As I pushed my disabled bicycle along, I noticed the guard jingling his keys in his right pocket.

There was a suspicious and certain rhythm to this jingling. As I approached, he was jingling even harder. He made no attempt to conceal his actions, and as I approached, he even began to moan like a porn star and deliberately looked me in the eye.

I can get a bit mouthy, but on this occasion, I had a flash of insight. It wouldn't be a good idea to get mouthy to a rifle-toting *and* masturbating soldier. So quite sensibly, I pushed my little bicycle past, carrying on my way towards town. I was a tad shaken up and disgusted, but not fearful.

I continued towards town. I pushed the bike along the road behind the 16th century fort built by the Portuguese and somewhat destroyed by the conflict. As I passed the fort, I spied a man urinating at the roadside. He also spied me but continued his business. Then, folding his penis back into his pants he called out, "Madame, where are you going?" Again, good sense prevailed, and I trundled along eyes front.

Finally, I was back in Jaffna town and began looking for Rio's ice-cream parlour. It took me about half an hour to find Point Pedro Road, a very long, industrial section of town where building supplies, hardware and plumbing supplies are sold. I pushed my bike to one end of the road. No ice cream parlour.

I asked for directions. Nobody seemed to understand me. I pushed my bike all the way to the other end. Still no ice-cream parlour. I asked for directions. Nobody seemed to understand me.

Bill and I had left home together. He had the knapsack with him, containing our phones, money and snacks. I didn't have a rupee to my name. I had no phone. I had no water. I didn't know Bill's cell phone number, as I had programmed it into my cell phone and therefore, had never bothered to memorise it. I carried no identification.

As the night gathered, I decided I had better just go home. I was dying of thirst, and dust coated my face. My bare legs were serving as a king's feast to dengue and malaria-carrying mosquitoes. I was concerned that Bill was worried, so I hurried my broken bike along in the direction of Chundikuli.

I arrived home at dusk. Bill's bicycle was in the yard, but he was not. Apparently, he had switched to the motorbike to look for me. I didn't have a key to the house, but luckily, Marcia was home and let me in.

Bill got home after spending a couple of hours driving around trying to find me. He had been worried, but not frantic. It was a good lesson for me in safety and preparedness.

At times, I lacked a sense of hyper vigilance, an awareness of my surroundings, and a mental notetaking of landmarks to secure a way home, as the world always seemed safe to me. Now, I developed a plan to ensure future safety. From that time on, I carried my own knapsack, I packed my own phone, I carried money and a house key with me.

I always carried identification. I drilled Bill's phone number into my brain. Soon after, another incident heightened my sense of vigilance and uneasiness.

4th February was Independence Day. Marcia and I scooted out to a restaurant called USA for their delicious prawn curry. As we were walking back, a deafening roar of engines startled us. From around the corner, a motorcycle gang blasted up the street, the sound reverberating inside our bodies. They tore down the street on huge black motorbikes with tires more suitable for a bush quad.

The dozen men, encased in black bulletproof vests, black padded pants that looked like armour, black army boots and black motorcycle helmets, had their faces hidden with black balaclava ski masks and goggles. They careened down the street in formation, like a gang of Hell's Angels. One of the men, seeing us standing petrified on the shoulder of the road, performed a wheelie, never breaking formation. The sound diminished as they rounded the corner and disappeared.

Shaken, but curious, we ventured into town to see what was happening. The merchants told us that there was going to be a parade with the President of Sri Lanka, Mahinda Rajapaksa, who was in town for a ribbon cutting. The street was fluttering with Sri Lankan flags.

The military and the police had ordered the Tamil people to display patriotism by flying Sinhala flags. It turned out that the motorcycle men were the bodyguards of the president. The volume, the size of the bikes and the men in their all-black costumes were a show of force, intimidation and power.

I could imagine how the Tamil people in Jaffna felt as the army, police and this squad of bodyguards descended upon them. The war had been over just for one year. For thirty years, a military presence held sway over the people who were demanding equal rights to education and employment.

The next week, I was conducting a group therapy session with the trauma team staff. When I started the group therapy training, I had established very strict boundaries within the team and with other staff members who were not in the group. The rules were that once I closed the training room door, we were not to be disturbed unless there was an emergency.

I emphasised that interruptions stop the flow of emotion while a client is telling a story, so intrusions had to be kept to a minimum. It took a long time for the outside staff to see the importance of privacy and safety in the counselling room, but after a while they understood not to disturb us for the hour of counselling.

However, a week after the President was in town, the staff outside the room began waving to me through the window, trying to get my attention. I ignored them, shaking my head. They continued jumping around and waving with worried looks on their faces. Then came a timid knock on the door. Annoyed, I excused myself and opened the door a crack.

"There is a soldier here, demanding to see Liniatha," the secretary informed me in a whisper.

A bit shaken, I called Liniatha forward, and she left with the uniformed Sri Lankan soldier. When the others in the team saw how shaken I was, they told me that they all could be subjected to interrogation in an effort for the army to obtain information about their clients. I began to feel less safe not only for myself but also for my Tamil friends and colleagues.

I was very upset about this military pressure for staff to disclose information gained from a counselling session. To protect my students, I reported this incident to my supervisor, Dr Sivayokan. He promised to speak to the chief of the military.

I knew this had been going on before I came and would continue after I left, but witnessing the power, control and manipulation made the war and the oppression of the people much more real to me. I felt vulnerable now.

Since the execution in Mexico, we felt a reactive impulse to drop to the ground when fireworks exploded in the frequent religious ceremonies here. Other than that, I had not felt vulnerable in Nuwara Eliya. In Jaffna I did, although I knew I was protected by my colour and privilege. I came to understand the feeling of vulnerability by people who lacked this protection and had suffered through fear, war and oppression.

As women, Jo, Beth, Mary and I experienced a taste of gender discrimination. The Security Forces Swimming Pool in the middle of town is open for women to swim on Thursdays from three to six o'clock. The other swim times were for the exclusive use of men.

So, on Thursdays, we VSO women headed to 1st Cross Street to the pool embedded in the grounds of Central College. The ticket man did double duty as a security guard, so men were prevented from entering the compound. A female lifeguard attired in a sari or a shalwar kept us safe from her deck chair as we swam our laps.

There were just two or three of us women in the pool at any given time. Very few Tamil women came for a swim. Bathing suits for women, it seemed, were not tolerated well by Tamil society. In both Tamil and Sinhala societies, sexual harassment is prevalent. Many of the VSO women who were in their mid to late thirties, had reported inappropriate sexual incidences on buses and on the streets. For a while I had not experienced any problem, but one Tuesday, as I cycled home for lunch, the chain broke on my bike forcing me to push it the rest of the way.

As I entered our lane, I saw that a man was standing there, leaning up against his bicycle. He was tall, thin, about twenty-twenty-five years old, well-groomed in a black and red golf shirt and black jeans. I thought his bike was a Lumala. He began squeezing his breast and pointing at my breast in a lewd manner.

"Fuck off," I said and kept walking. He hopped on his bike and cycled ahead of me into my side lane. I stopped walking and attempted to phone Bill, who was at home at the end of the lane. However, sunlight was shining on the phone display preventing me from reading the numbers programmed into the phone.

The man cycled back out of the side lane. Believing he had been scared off, I entered the lane to race toward my home. Instead of leaving, he followed on his bicycle, passed me, turned around and stopped his bike right in front of me. He began squeezing his breast again. I yelled and swore at him again. He tried to grab my breast as I tried to pass.

I kept walking, pushing my bike and scooted inside my gate. I hollered at Bill. He rushed out and I told him what had happened. Arming himself with a broomstick, he ran out in search, but the man had disappeared. What was most disconcerting was that the man appeared to know where I lived, and he was not intimidated by my shouting.

My organisation insisted on me making a police report. At the police station, despite a long line of dishevelled and tired looking men and women, 'Dr Nordick' was hustled to the front of the line and then ushered in to see the Chief Inspector of the Jaffna Police Department. Clad in running shorts and T-shirt, the Chief apologised for the man's behaviour, gave me his personal cell phone numbers, advised me to call him at any time should I feel unsafe and assured me that they take this type of 'crime' very seriously.

He wasn't much interested in the description of the man or the map that I had drawn. He finally directed a duty officer to take my statement, which I had brought with me. The officer began tearing off the margins of my statement and then glued my written statement into his large notebook. I was given file number CIB 2/40/65I and dismissed with a handshake and another apology on behalf of Sri Lankan men.

A month later, to the day, I encountered the man again. I was on my way home for lunch when the man on his bicycle passed me as I rode along Colombothurai Road. He rode very slowly in front of me, causing me to pass him. He followed me along Colombothurai Road and then onto Vidhans Lane. There, he sped up, and as he passed me, ran his hand up along my entire back, from buttocks to shoulder.

"Fuck off," I swore at him, hoping to alert a neighbour. He cycled past me but continued to make hand gestures as if he was still stroking my back. I peddled home with uncharacteristic speed.

176

I was convinced it was the same man. He was in his early twenties, had on an orange and black striped shirt, had black pants, rode a Lumala bike and again, did not speak and was not threatened or concerned about the ruckus my shouting created in the quiet neighbourhood.

I doubted there was any way he had been watching for me, as my routine was too varied. I didn't always go home for lunch, nor did I always go at the same time, and I was often on my motorcycle rather than my bike. I believed that he was an opportunist. I wrote to the Chief of Police about the second incident—just to get it documented in case he showed up again.

By this time, I had to repeat my story many times over. I was beginning to formulate a pretty good idea about what it must be like for a woman who was violated; repeating the story over and over to strangers, pointing to body parts in a society where sexual body parts are not acknowledged, never mind mentioned.

I began to understand what being violated might mean in a culture where being touched meant you might not receive a marriage proposal, which is the source of economic security for many women. I became aware that this type of incident was underreported. Even I felt a bit powerless by the end of it all and became more wary and vigilant on the streets.

Chapter 26
More Than a Birthday Surprise

It is interesting how people who hate cats forget this when they get one.

As we turned the calendar to February, I realised Bill's birthday was approaching. My husband was turning seventy! He was getting old! To cheer him up, Marcia and I began scheming a big surprise party.

The weekend of 4 February was a holiday weekend in Sri Lanka, thus allowing our VSO colleagues from Colombo, Kandy, Puttalam and Batticaloa time to attend the party. We sent out invitations and arranged beds. Between Jo, Mary, Marcia and Bill and I, we had just enough beds, couches and mats to bed everyone down for the night.

The day of the party, Bill was impossible to get out of the house. He didn't feel like doing anything. He was too tired to go for a bike ride. He was disinterested in a swim. We resorted to decorating Marcia's suite upstairs for the party. Most of the guests had arrived by that time, and nearly twenty people had slipped past our door and tiptoed up the outside stairs to Marcia's suite.

Marcia and I contrived to get Bill a special birthday present. The large rats that entered our house at night prompted us to find the perfect gift for him. These shaggy rats wiggled into the house through holes in the sink and the bathroom water drain.

Bill had exterminated three of them so far, but it was a grisly job. Mousetraps sold in the Jaffna shops were sticky pads sodden with glue. The rats, trapped in the glue, would remain there until Bill covered them with a plastic bag and beat them to death with a broom. It was very gruesome, especially if we were away all week while a rat was decomposing into the glue.

We wanted to spare Bill more killing, so Marcia and I decided to secure a cat to help with the rat problem. Marcia put the word out through the expat grapevine, and within a week, she got a call from her French teacher, Gerard.

"Gerard has found a cat for us," Marcia exclaimed, flying down the stairs. "He wants to know if we can come and see it after work."

We were so excited! After work Marcia and I donned our motorcycle helmets, hopped on our scooters and headed down Kachcheri Nallur Road to Gerard's office. Large leafy trees canopied the grounds, and a menagerie of small animals sat in cages or roamed the yard. These animals had all been rescued by Gerard or his security personnel from certain starvation and injury.

Gerard led us out to the compound. The dirt yard was enclosed with a fence, and sunshine dappled through the large trees. A small cage sat in a shaded corner of the yard. Gerard opened the cage and lifted a small scrap of fabric.

Marcia and I both gasped. Nestled into the fabric was a tiny orange kitten, no more than a couple of weeks old, eyes still half glued shut. The scrawny, bald kitten was mewling at the top of its underdeveloped lungs, its tiny feet pawing at the air.

The end of its tiny tail was bent, like it had been broken and it was wet from the kitten sucking on it. He was being bottle-fed cow's milk by Gerard's security staff.

"Gee, I don't know," I said, looking at Marcia with dismay. "He's so tiny. It'll be a long time until he can mouse."

Marcia nodded in agreement, yet her eyes were shining, encouraging me. I hemmed and hawed, but I knew I would have to take this baby home, as a situation that took place when we had first arrived in Jaffna still haunted me.

About two days after arriving in Jaffna, Marcia and I were walking back to the Thinakkural Rest Guest House from our orientation and cut through an alley. There in the alley were two roly-poly puppies, one black, the other with brown and white patches, barely able to walk and with no mother in sight. They stumbled about in the grass, then onto the road.

Marcia was overcome. Upset at the danger these tiny creatures were in, she moaned, "We should take them home."

"No, Marcia, we can't. We can't look after dogs here. And what are we to do with them when we go home? Don't do it," I warned her, but I was sick at heart too. We turned our backs on the little babies and hurried home, feeling guilty and hoping the mother was around somewhere.

The next day, we cut through the alley again. We shouldn't have. The little brown puppy with the brown and white patches had been hit by a trishaw and lay tiny, abandoned and dead in the alley. The black puppy licked at his sibling, whimpering. We avoided the alley after that until a week or so later. By then, both puppies were gone.

"Yes, I will take him," I blurted out, remembering the two puppies we left in the alley to die. Marcia immediately christened him Judge. Lucky for us, Gerard agreed to keep him until the night of the party.

At the party, following the SURPRISE! SURPRISE! Bill was handed a small orange plastic basket with a bright birthday bow tied to it. He lifted off the lid and Judge's little bedraggled head emerged. Bill seemed stunned.

"Oh," he said. Then a startled, "Oh." Then, "Oh," in disbelief as he sought me out to see if I had participated in this gift, a gift that knew came with responsibility. I nodded, avoiding his eyes.

That night, we drank wine and feasted on birthday cake. Music from our tiny speakers poured into the warm garden. Dancing broke out. Later, everyone moved outdoors to visit quietly and trace the full moon as it travelled the night sky.

In the wee hours of the morning, Bill and I climbed in under the mosquito net, exhausted. We closed our eyes. "Meew, meew." Tiny, pathetic sounds emerged from the orange basket we had placed near our bed. We both sat bolt upright.

The mewing was escalating in volume and frequency, making us anxious. Gerard had supplied us with a tiny baby bottle and some human baby formula for feeding. We made up a bottle for Judge as quickly as possible, and Bill sat down to feed him.

Hysterical for food, he clawed at Bill's hand. I wrapped Bill's hand in a small hand towel, and Judge managed to latch onto the bottle's nipple. While he sucked, he began kneading his sharp little claws into the cloth that held Bill's bleeding hand. Bill then placed him back into the plastic basket lined with a soft towel. Judge snuggled in and slept all night.

As he came to trust regular mealtimes, sunshine and a tender master, Judge started to settle. He was happy, rambunctious, mischievous and sweet. He gave us pure joy, reducing our homesickness. He also grew in strength.

His hair filled in. He toilet trained, flinging sand all over the place in his sweet earnestness to cover his waste. He romped and tumbled and made us laugh so much. He loved rolling in the sunshine on the dirt driveway, flipping back and forth, back and forth.

Judgey was a source of entertainment but was also a hassle for us. One day, as I came home from work, Bill met me at the gate in a panic. "Come here," he said, dragging me over to the jackfruit tree. "Look!"

We stretched our necks, and I spied Judgey near the top of the leafy, thirty-foot tree. Claws sunk into the bark of a skinny branch, he was looking down at us in helplessness. He must have been there for hours. Fear gripped me.

"Come on, Judgey, I am here," I coaxed. Bill stood on the roots of the tree, balancing himself with one hand. He stretched his other arm up towards Judge, splaying his hand to create a vessel for him to climb to safety.

Judge seemed to realise that Bill was trying to rescue him. He made many attempts to move down the tree but kept retreating to the twiggy branch when the descent became too frightening.

Aggressive black crows swarmed, and sensing a dinner, swooped, threatening to pluck him out of the tree. Outraged, we snatched rocks from the garden and pelted them. The birds, annoyed and squawking, flew off. We were beside ourselves and it was getting dark.

Bill's problem-solving skills kicked in. He ran to the house and returned with a huge roll of duct tape. From the back of the house, he retrieved a rake. He hollered, "Collect long sticks from the yard."

As I ran around collecting sticks, he extended our reach by duct taping the sticks in sections to the homemade rake. The stick handle was now fifteen feet long. Then, he slapped canned cat food onto the rake head.

The stick handle curved but held as he lifted the rake high into the tree. Lured by the food, Judge moved part way down the tree but was still unable to climb down the most vertical part of the trunk. Bill hurried to the back of the house where he found an eight-foot plank about four inches wide.

He propped the plank against the tree trunk, forming a ramp to help Judge down the last, branchless section. As he neared the ground, Bill grabbed him, scolded him and then buried his face into his neck to hide tears of relief.

Judge darted into the kitchen where his food and water sat in stainless steel bowls on the floor. He purred as he ate. We watched, in relief, our arms around each other wondering how this tiny, gangly ginger kitten had become so precious.

He had somehow become a symbol of our children, bequeathing upon us a living creature to nourish, cherish, protect and parent. The inability to protect him would have destroyed us.

Real danger did, however, exist for Judge in our yard. Our home in Jaffna had a small cobra den situated at the base of our huge jackfruit tree. Cobras, called *naya* in Sinhala, are territorial, and often found near human habitations. We never did see any cobras ourselves, but one day a man clearing the empty lot next door was startled by one.

Another critter patrolled our yard as well. I saw the creature moving in the grass near the vegetable pit. He looked at me, and I looked at him. It was unnerving to be stared down by a creature with red eyes and a flaring red nose. He seemed sinister. I googled it and found out it was a mongoose.

There are four types of mongoose in Sri Lanka. Our resident mongoose was a grey mongoose about the size of a house cat, but with a much longer nose and tail. Most mornings, it scooted along our garden wall, crawled down a tree near the wall and slunk over to our vegetable scrap pit.

There, at the depression in the earth filled daily with our potato peels, carrot peelings and apple cores, the mongoose feasted. Then, it disappeared and reappeared at dusk, patrolling the outer edges of the yard. We liked to think it ate the cobra that lived in the den.

The mongoose never made a sound and was never aggressive. I began to trust it and look forward to its arrival each day. That was until we got Judgey. One evening the mongoose appeared at the vegetable pit. Judge flew over to the pit before we could stop her. She danced around the pit, trying to get the attention of the mongoose. Bill declared in astonishment, "They are friends!"

Sure enough, Judge was making sweet overtures to play. However, the mongoose was disinterested in Judge, preferring our composting vegetables to an orange furball. I didn't worry about the mongoose after that.

Judge grew on us quickly. She gave Bill meaning and purpose and company for the long hours while I was at work. She also gave us something we didn't even know we needed. Living far from friends and family, in isolation, in a different country, Judge provided us some reprieve from the intensity of sharing a life that had limited input from the outside world. We became a family triangle.

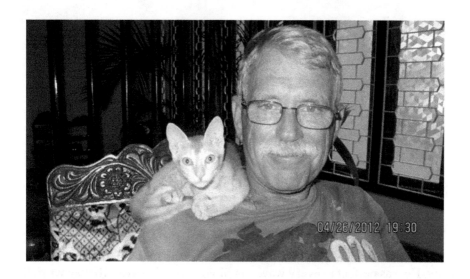

Bill and his growing 70th birthday present, an abandoned kitten

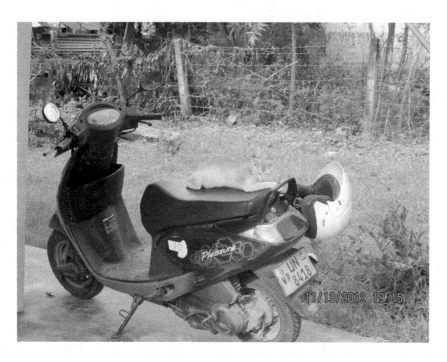

Judgey making herself at home on the VSO scooter

Chapter 27
Grannying from Afar

I pray for the gift of bilocation. I want to be here and I want to be there – at the same time. I struggle with this temporal limitation.

In March, we were gifted with the arrival of a new grandson, Mickey Ryan Finley. He was perfect in every way. Via Skype, we witnessed Mickey wriggling and squeezing his daddy's fingers from his home in Calgary. He blinked and stayed awake during the entire call.

His dad took off his booties and exposed his long toes and big feet to us. We were thrilled. We also knew that two more grandchildren were on their way. It was hard for me to be so far away from our children, especially as they started their families. Our family was changing.

Bill seemed to be undergoing some radical change as well. He had lived a conservative life since becoming a judge. Decorum, diplomacy, and dignity governed him. He hadn't always been staid, but since I'd met him, he had lived a life suitable to his position. However, after years of conservatism, he began growing his greying blonde hair and beard.

At first, I didn't know if I liked his new look or not. The beard was through the worst of the growing out stage, but for a few days, I couldn't even look at him. He reminded me of my dad when he was too tired and old to shave. His hair, too, became unruly and as it did, he began to run his hands through it more often, making it stick up and out.

I tried to ignore the change. Then, one day, a few weeks later, he sauntered out of the bathroom. His beard was gone. Now he had a goatee. The changes in him made me realise that he too was shedding some old skin placed upon him by convention. I was glad for him but lamented the clean-cut man I had married.

Judge transformed too. As he grew, we began staring at his genitals. "I'm not so sure he is a boy," said Bill, concerned, lifting his tail and peering at his backside. It didn't seem as if there were any testicles or a penis, but he was so small it was hard to tell. Mary had a peek under the tail. "Judgey is a girl," she declared lowering the tail, giving Judge back her dignity.

Soon after, a long-anticipated phone call came. "I think I am in labour, Mom," my daughter Tanya gasped into the phone. "Contractions are coming seven to eight minutes apart."

A little later, she called me again. "Mom, I'm at the hospital, two centimetres dilated, baby fully effaced. Still a while to go. Baby doing great."

As it was late in Sri Lanka, I told Tanya that I was going to bed but to phone anytime. I awoke with a start at 1:30 a.m. Sri Lanka time. There had been no phone call. I called my sister, Teresa, who lived in the same town and had been like a second mother to Tanya.

She advised me that due to the slow progression of the labour, the nursery staff had dispatched everyone home, except Tanya and Brent. They were instructed to turn off their phones and get some sleep.

I went back to bed and slept fitfully. By morning, I had heard nothing. In a bit of panic, I telephoned the Nelson Hospital and asked to be transferred to the labour room. To my surprise, Tanya's doctor picked up the phone. I introduced myself. "Hello, I am Tanya Holowaychuk's Mom."

"We have been expecting you," he chattered. "Skype is set up and all is well, although I may have to do a C-section if she doesn't move along soon. She has been in labour more than thirty hours."

Via a very poor Internet connection, Teresa stood in as Tanya's doula and continued a tense but newsy communication. We persevered through dropped calls, poor video quality, garbled voices and frozen screens as the birth progressed. I had one small opportunity to offer Tanya love and encouragement before she was taken to the operating room.

Then I waited and waited. Nothing, nothing, nothing. Then my sister came back on Skype. "It's a boy!" she exclaimed. "He is 7 lbs, 14 ounces of perfection!"

With Skype, I saw that little man, Michael Gary, feasting on breast milk, giving gaseous grins, splaying his giant fingers and snoozing in his mother's arms. He became our fifth grandchild and the newest cousin for Jayden, Lainee, Gwendylen and Mickey, our other grandchildren.

On 17 August, another granddaughter of ours slipped into the world. She was a week overdue, languishing in the womb. She was tiny and beautiful. Thanks to technology, I got play-by-play updates via text.

Richard: On way to hospital. They are inducing Julie at 5:30 p.m.

Grandma: Oh, wonderful. We will have a little girl today. I love U. Give our love to Julie. Call when she is settled in. Love. Mom.

Richard: Eight centimetres right now.

Grandma: Oh, wow, going along quickly then. How is she doing? How are you doing?

Richard: Mega pain, getting drugs. I want to go home.

Grandma: You stay right where you are. No time for cowardice! She needs U strong.

Richard: I was kidding, Mom.

Grandma: I know, so was I.

Richard: 10:35 p.m., she's out and she looks good! Say hello to Penelope Lily Frances!

Grandma: Congratulations, Son. Well done, you two!

I had decided to call this little flower Poppy, as a nickname. When I sent out my blog, I included a bright red poppy to depict her. Unbeknownst to me, her parents had already planned to call her Poppy. It was serendipitous.

I was excited for a new grandbaby and relieved that all had gone well, but couldn't seem to hold back a tidal wave of loss that seeped in. I felt forlorn. I was not there to hold my new grandchildren and to assist these children of ours who were now new parents. I remembered all too well the difficult few months of sleep deprivation that dogged me after the births of my own children.

Our children still needed our support. What were we doing in Sri Lanka when we had so many responsibilities at home? Guilt and longing were crushing me.

My homesickness made me count the days until I could go home. Both Bill and I were struggling. We missed big things like our treasured family. I missed my good Mom, whom I had left just ten days after the loss of her husband of sixty years.

I missed my four sisters and my three brothers and my numerous nieces and nephews. We missed our friends with whom we enjoyed hiking, cycling, golfing and camping.

We missed little things like going out for a great steak and jumping into our little Miata sports car for a Sunday car ride. We missed a movie at the theatre. We missed playing whist and other card games whilst crunching Lays potato chips. Bill missed his weekly bridge match.

We missed the beauty and bleakness of Lac du Bois where we hiked, and we missed the joy of family gatherings at Kamloops Lake. Two years away from home was much harder than we had ever dreamed.

We were ready to go home, but we had a job to do that was not finished. We had made a commitment, and we were determined to see it through. I rarely took something on without completing. Time was speeding along, but weirdly, daily life seemed to drag.

I didn't feel as grateful for the CUSO/VSO opportunity as it now interfered with my desire to go home. Although, each time we discussed going home, we both agreed we weren't quitters.

Chapter 28
Our Luck Running Out

Luck isn't manifested. It is a divine gift.

The honeymoon we experienced with the country was well over, and we began to think we were jinxed. We had another motorbike crash. One Sunday, after swimming at Casurina Beach, we headed back into the crowded mayhem of Jaffna City traffic.

It had been a great day. The sun was warm on our faces and the light breeze blowing about our clothing cooled us as we rode our scooter home. We rounded a corner, but a minibus was parked too close. The next thing we knew, my helmet was plastered into the side of the minivan and our bike followed.

"Bill, what happened?" I inquired as I disentangled myself from under the bike, shaken but not hurt.

"I don't know," Bill moaned. Upset, he dismounted and sheepishly removed his helmet.

A crowd had gathered. Bill told the people in English that he was responsible, and a young lad tore off to find the driver of the vehicle. A dozen men began inspecting the dent on the side of the minivan, still loaded with passengers. Bill was flustered and embarrassed and used his only Tamil word repeatedly— Nandri. Nandri. Thank you. Thank you.

One old biddy inside the bus hung her toothless old face out the window, cackling and grinning at our misfortune. Over and over, she cackled to the driver, who had arrived by then to assess the damage, "Money, Money." Cackle, cackle.

I wanted to strangle her. The men ran their hands over the damage, shaking their heads. They seemed unable to agree on the cause of the accident and damages owing.

An older man, barefoot and sarong-clad, sauntered over to the raucous crowd. He raised his arms. The people silenced. He spoke, and we assumed he gave his rendition of the accident to the crowd.

He pointed out that the minibus was too close to the corner and parked more on the road than on the side of the road. In addition, and to our astonishment, he pointed to a large pothole in the road where we had tipped the bike. We hadn't even realised that we'd plunged our bike into the pothole. The people listened to his sage wisdom.

"How much? How much?" Bill asked, holding out his open wallet to demonstrate his willingness to rectify his mistake.

With much debating back and forth, the men again ran their hands over the dents and scratches of the bus. A verdict was reached. One thousand Sri Lankan rupees (about $50) should cover the damage.

"Are you sure that is enough?" Bill asked in growing concern. "I can pay more," declared the judicious Mr Blair. "Nandri, nandri." I wanted to kick him.

Fishing out a five thousand rupee note, Bill handed it over to the driver, and someone secured him appropriate change. The transaction completed, we donned our helmets and scuttled off to the grocery store. Bill was shaken up, now believing he was getting too old to drive the scooter.

I was beginning to wonder the same, but a man in the grocery store told Bill he had witnessed our incident. He believed the bus was parked too close to a corner, and the crash wasn't our fault. We felt better.

However, not much later, one of our excursions turned very dangerous. We had decided to head out for a hike and a swim to Kayts Island. We set off in two groups: Bill, Jo, Mary and I hopped in the Toyota, while Mischi and Marcia planned to join us later at the beach.

We explored a region that meandered past a small village east of Chetty Beach and walked in the jungle that followed the coastline. Up until 2010, the area was deemed a high security zone and had been laid flat by the tsunami that wiped out the homes along the northern coast. The jungle was dotted with abandoned homes, their foundations now rubble and thick with garbage.

Each crumbling home had a well nearby. The wells were deep holes in the ground, some as much as twenty feet deep. Some of the wells were filled to the brim with water while in others the water levels had receded, and water reflected from far below. The wells had absolutely no siding on them; the edges of the opening were flush with the ground.

Continuing our hike and enjoying the building of the morning heat, we passed a construction site where a group of men were rebuilding one of the homes. They waved and stared at the novelty of four foreigners hiking in their village. Young Tamil children began to follow us, skulking behind bushes whenever we looked back. We hollered at them to join us, but they disappeared into the brush.

We discovered a grassy knoll along the beach, a perfect place for our picnic lunch. We stretched out on the grass and munched fresh mangosteens and Scan Jumbo peanuts. We sunned on the bank then hiked back along the abandoned trail through the palmyra forest, heading for Chetty Beach to meet up with Mischi and Marcia.

However, Mischi and Marcia were not at Chetty Beach. An hour passed and then another. We were preparing to head home when they finally arrived, led by Mischi's two white doggies, Mia and Blanca. The story of why they were late tumbled out of them.

They had arrived in the little village not long after us and decided to catch up with us. They passed the spot where the men were constructing the house, and as they made their way through the jungle, Mia darted off chasing a ground squirrel. Her frolic turned into a nightmare as she leaped into one of those deep-water wells.

In fright, her mother, Blanca followed in after her. Seeing his little doggies panicking in the dark water far below, Mischi jumped in to save them. He thought that he would be able to stand in the well, but the water was too deep.

The dogs pawed at Mischi, scratching him as they tried to gain traction on his shoulders. Mischi struggled to keep himself afloat. He realised his small dogs wouldn't last long in the freezing cold water and neither would he.

The steep walls of the well were slippery and sheer, with no supports or crevices to take hold. Marcia was shocked to see her partner and his two little dogs struggling to stay afloat in a deep dark well in the middle of the Jaffna jungle.

"Go and get help! And get the kite from the van too," Mischi yelled. He was a renowned kite surfer in Sri Lanka and operated his own kite surfing school in Putalaam.

Marcia ran to the construction site, where she tried to make her plight known to the men working on the house. Marcia spoke no Tamil and relied on English and sign language to communicate the urgency. "Help, I need help," she pleaded. They didn't understand. She gestured in a swimming motion. They didn't understand. She used her hand to mimic cutting her throat. They didn't understand her and made no attempts to come to her rescue.

Feeling it was futile to continue, she raced towards their Volkswagen, grateful they hadn't locked the vehicle as the keys were in Mischi's swimming trunks deep down in the well. She flung open the back hatch, grabbed Mischi's kite and ran back to the well. Following Mischi's instructions, Marcia threw down an edge of the kite and held fast to the point of the triangle.

Mischi was able to get some relief as he clung to the kite. By then, he had been treading for more than fifteen minutes in the icy water.

After many failed attempts, Mischi, using the kite for balance and stability, was able to brace his legs against the curved wall of the well. He then straightened his legs and pressed his back up against the opposite side. Once in position, he placed the dogs on his lap.

Moving with caution, he shifted his feet an inch upward and then heaved his back up the wall an inch or two. Using all his strength, he 'walked' out of the well with Marcia dragging the kite towards her as much as possible.

They were shaken from their experience, and we were all stunned by the gravity of the incident. We all realised the potential of a very different outcome. We felt gratitude that we were hugging our friends and not dealing with a tragedy. The burgeoning homesickness made us realise how far away from home we were.

Soon, another trouble arose. I was insane with an itch on my back and pubic area, especially at night. However, there was nothing to see. No rash, no redness, no lumps, no bumps. The itch seemed hidden, buried beneath in the subcutaneous layers of my skin.

I scratched until the itchy areas were raw. I was like the dogs on the street, going mad with the itch.

I sought a doctor and I had to take a blood test. I was diagnosed with an allergy and given antihistamines and hydrocortisone cream. I was still scratching on 15 September and went back to the doctor. I was treated for worms. On 30 September, I went back to the doctor who repeated the blood tests. Apparently, there was a 'slight viral picture', and I was given more antihistamines.

The itching continued, so I marched back to the doctor. He referred me to a dermatologist. By then, small red spots had appeared on my back. After taking my history and examining me, the dermatologist opined the spots were 'consistent with scabies'.

Scabies is caused by a parasitic eight-legged mite that burrows into the skin, causing intense itching. I had no idea how I got it as it requires prolonged skin to skin contact and Bill didn't have them. By the time I got treatment, my bites were beginning to dry up, but Bill was, by then, tearing off his skin. The dermatologist offered to treat both of us with a cream called Permethrin.

I felt the dermatologist's inclusion of some treatment for Bill was unfair. First, he wasn't even at the doctor's office and secondly, he received prompt and immediate treatment, whilst I had endured the parasitic burrowing for six weeks. Bill, undisturbed by the inequality of the situation, grabbed at his prescription cream and liberally applied the medication. The symptoms improved within the week.

My friend Marlene, after reading about the sexual assaults, the accidents and the scabies wrote to me, "Your luck is running out. It is time to come home." I was beginning to feel that maybe she was right.

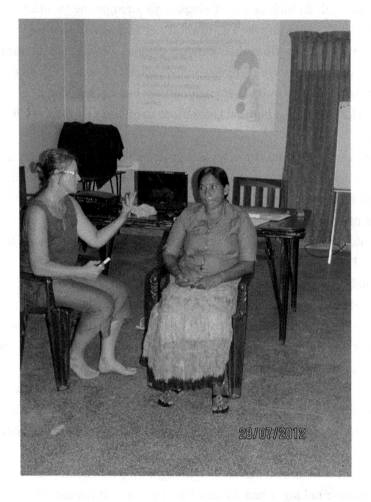

Teaching Communication skills to community support workers in Jaffna

Chapter 29
Two Very Different Celebrations

There is something innate about celebration and ritual.
They permeate all cultures.

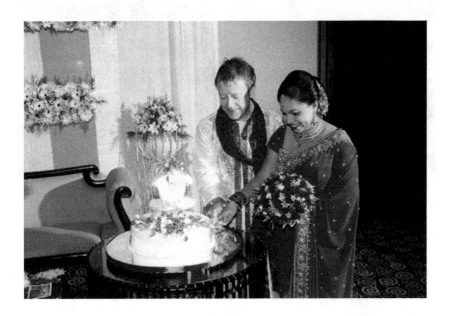

Mark and Sewwandi Chamberlain's wedding in Colombo

Many good things were still happening. In May, our fellow VSO colleague, Mark, married his Sri Lankan sweetheart, Sewwandi. Mark was from Britain and was a mental health nurse working in Kandy. He had met and fallen in love with Sewwandi in Colombo after being introduced by Marjorie.

Mark and Sewwandi invited all the VSO volunteers to the wedding celebration in Colombo. Careful organisation with the VSO Sri Lanka office enabled us to coordinate the wedding with one of our regular sector group meetings.

The September wedding day was a big event for all VSO volunteers. In preparation for the event, the Jaffna VSO women went on a sari shopping expedition and in the end, we all looked like Jaffna parrots—bright and colourful! Sewwandi had scheduled a cosmetologist to do the 'dressing' for us, which involved a total of fourteen safety pins and an underskirt to perfect a sari wrap.

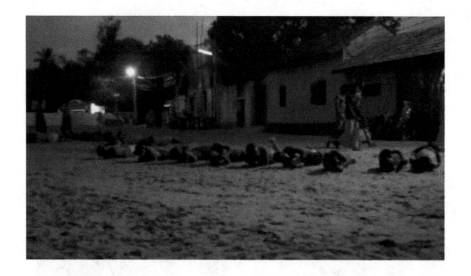

Hindu men in devotion rolling around Nallur Temple at dawn

Our hair was coiffed by a stylist and finally we were ready for the one-hour van ride to the reception hall. The bride and groom served cake, copious amounts of wine and good gin, fed us well and requested that the band play some western and Sinhala music.

Bill was delighted. With his long hair and sarong, combined with his lust for dancing, he rocked the dance floor. Coupled with a lack of dancing opportunities for the past two years and good music, Bill danced *every* dance with his somewhat reluctant partner.

The highlight of his dancing included showing off his country two-step to a Sri Lankan singer crooning Dwight Yoakam's *Crazy Little Thing Called Love*. We were happy. We knew this might be the last time all the VSO volunteers would be together in Sri Lanka.

A couple of months later, we took part in a very different kind of celebration. The Ther Festival is Jaffna's Nallur Kandaswamy Temple's annual twenty-five-day festival. Considered to be the grandest and most venerated Hindu festival in

194

Sri Lanka, it is held during the months of August or September depending on the temple calendar.

The local community of Jaffna is joined by thousands of Sri Lankan Tamils and Tamil diaspora who flock to the temple during the festival to worship Lord Murugan. Devotees attend the daily puja ceremonies during the early morning and again in the evenings. Puja is a form of devotional worship to the deities of Hinduism.

I went alone, to take in the puja ceremonies, camera in hand. I arrived in the dark and peered in disbelief through the bars of the wrought iron fencing around the temple. The events I saw gave meaning to the term 'holy rollers' and made me wonder if this might be the origin of that expression.

About fifty bare-chested men, wrapped in sarongs they had tucked between their legs, or in loin cloths, rolled in the dirt around the entire perimeter of the huge temple. With their arms either crossed over their bare chests or stretched out above their heads, they made two rounds: one around the inside of the temple and one around the outside of the temple for the entire twenty-five days.

They were sweating and exhausted, but continued to roll, shouting, "A-ro-ha-ra, A-ro-ha-ra." It left me emotional to see such religious devotion and fervour.

The women's puja was different, but just as exhausting. They also moved around the entire temple grounds, but in their form of devotion, they took three to four steps and then knelt and lowered themselves into a full bow, forehead to the ground. Then, they arose and took another three to four steps and knelt.

They made their way around the temple kneeling and stepping. They all looked tired, and I heard that some people perform their puja for several hours every day.

On the final round, the men were given a coconut by a support person to carry as they rolled into the temple, kissing a brass plate at the door as they crossed the threshold. As they left the temple, they smashed the coconut by dashing it to the ground. Watery coconut milk bled onto the pavement.

Inside the temple, people milled around, had their breakfast, meditated and worshipped in front of the many gods present. They burned incense. Sinhala policemen provided security for the event. In deference to temple rules, the policemen had removed their shirts. It was distracting.

I was fascinated. The festival was breath-taking and beautiful, but foreign. After watching until dawn, I jumped back on my bike and cycled home. I couldn't wait to tell Bill and the others what they had missed. The following morning, the entire Jaffna Family pulled themselves out of bed to go and watch the ceremonies.

We entered the gates of the temple yard. Our eyes bugged. Devotees were practicing mortification. Some were arriving on foot with skewers through the flesh of their backs or chests to honour the gods or to repay a favour from the gods. Others arrived dangling face down from a mast mounted on pickup trucks and tractors.

Their bodies were held by ropes attached to large skewers that pierced their backs like shish kabobs. Large meat hooks were then hooked into the back of their thighs. It was horrible and fascinating to watch the young men dangling by their skin, like a log ready to be placed on a timber pile.

The grounds became crowded with bare-chested men, brightly dressed women and children, all barefoot. An enormous chariot adorned with four statues of rearing and pawing white horses was pushed out into the temple yard. The fifty-foot chariot had two attached ropes capable of securing an ocean liner.

Thousands of the shirtless men, young and old, hoisted the ropes upon their shoulders and began pulling at the chariot, like a mighty tug of war. I noticed that many of the men had healed scarring upon their bodies from skewering in previous festivals.

The ropes became taut, and the crowd swelled. The men leaned into the ropes and the chariot begrudgingly released its inertia and lumbered forward. It felt dangerous in the crush of the crowd, our footing unbalanced and erratic, our bodies forced to move with the pressure of the crowd.

I worried about being trampled as the chariot lumbered into the mass of people. It was exhilarating and terrifying at the same time.

The Jaffna Family linked arms and inched towards the exit of the temple grounds. Once at the gate, we exited in a rush to avoid being squashed by the press of people. Brushing the dust from our clothes, we trudged down Temple Road to Maria's Guest House for a cold beer and reflections on what had just taken place.

I marvelled at the devotion and the rich rituals of the Hindu people, but I was deeply impacted by the thrill of a possible crush from the chariot or a possible trampling from the crowd. This sensation of being on a precipice and balancing between thrill and danger has never left me.

Chapter 30
Lessons Learned on Bed 9

Getting sick makes me realize only one thing. I don't want to get sick.

I loved my work. It was rewarding to see the skills of the therapists I was training emerge, to see the organisation begin to see the rationale for change. Marcia was working hard to achieve some structural reorganisation. During the war, international NGOs poured money into local organisations for staff to provide therapy and counselling for the war affected.

However, since the war had ended, NGOs were more selective in their granting of funding. They now required organisations seeking funding to write funding proposals, provide timelines, measurable outcomes and fiscal accountability. Marcia feared that without training on how to write proposals and develop potential budgets with realistic costs, Shanthiham would be unable to compete for funding with other, more sophisticated organisations.

It was a difficult task as the management staff did not have the skills or the ability, so she enlisted my support to assist with the meetings and proposal writing.

I agreed to help, but soon it became clear that my bad luck was back. On 5 September 2012, I ended up in the hospital. It started rather strangely. I woke up on a Tuesday morning, feeling right as rain.

I sat down to consume my breakfast of buffalo curd and chopped papaya, and without warning my bowels gurgled, then liquefied and I sped to the bathroom. I decided to stay home from work as the diarrhoea and hideous cramping continued all day.

On Wednesday, I decided that I had regained some control over the problem, and so, returned to work. However, the vicious cramping and diarrhoea had not abated, and it was embarrassing to be running to the toilet at work. All the NGO staff shared just one bathroom, and I was embarrassed about the smells and the sounds that I emitted.

Shortly after lunch, the cramps intensified. I thought I was delivering a baby. I fled to the bathroom again and upon returning to my desk, Marcia lifted her head with concern.

"Are you alright?" She asked. To my surprise, I shook my head and started to cry. "I'm taking you home right now," Marcia declared, closing her computer and striding over to my desk to help me up. I felt incapable of driving my scooter home, so Marcia doubled me home on hers. She helped me hobble across the living room, settled me on my couch and hurried back to work.

Bill was out of town on a field trip with his English students. I was alone in the house with my orange cat. He sat on my chest, peering inquisitively at me. I began vomiting and running a fever. The cramping was severe.

Later that afternoon, Marcia came home from work and popped her head in the door. I was on the couch, miserable under a blanket. I couldn't move. Thoughtfully, she made peppermint tea, but my nausea was so intense I couldn't think of touching it.

Finally, Bill called from his field trip. "Bill, I think you need to take me to the hospital," I moaned into the phone.

"What? Okay, I will be there in a few minutes." Bill flew in the door and shouted like a boy scout taking charge on a wilderness outing. "I have a motorcycle waiting. One of my students can take you."

"I can't ride a scooter right now. I don't think I can sit up," I moaned from the couch. I could see his anxiety rising.

"Okay, I will go and find a trishaw." He rushed out of our blue garden gate, ran down Vidhans Lane and flagged down a trishaw on Colombothurai Road. He hopped in and instructed the driver to our yard. He held up a flat palm to the driver, instructing him in his own version of sign language to wait.

He rushed into the living room to help me stumble out the door into the yard. I somehow climbed into the backseat of the trishaw and gripped the black chrome bar that framed the driver's seat in front of me.

The driver, realising his passenger was ill and might vomit in his vehicle that provided him a livelihood, sped along to the Inpatient/Outpatient Department of a little clinic on Beach Road facing the watery bird-filled lagoon that surrounds Jaffna. Nursing sisters ran the clinic. I moaned as my head dangled over my lap, my body in turmoil.

Bill helped me into the clinic, and I sat like a drunk, waiting to be seen. The clinic had a file on me, as I had been there a month earlier when I was diagnosed with scabies.

Soon, a very aloof physician peppered me with questions about my symptoms, assessed me and then, unable to determine a diagnosis, declared I required hospital admission. However, the nursing Sister who was also present squared herself and set her jaw firm.

"Doctor, we have no beds," she informed him.

Cowed, the doctor turned to me and said, "You should go to the private hospital."

"No," I declared, feisty, despite my condition. "I don't want to go to the private hospital." The doctor looked at me like I had two heads. "I want to go to the government hospital," I said doubling over as another wave of cramping folded my intestines in half.

I was not in Sri Lanka to perpetuate colonialism and elitism. I wanted to be treated the same as my colleagues and the people of Sri Lanka.

Shrugging, he resigned from further discouragement. "Then, Madame, you will have to go to the admissions department of the Jaffna Teaching Hospital." He turned to the next patient, washing his hands of the foreign woman.

After a ten-minute bumpy trishaw ride, I dragged myself into the hospital and just lay on the concrete floor of the admissions room. I was aware that I was behaving like a baby, but I felt so rough. I take pride in being fit, strong and stoic.

Once seen, I was admitted with very little paperwork. Bill accompanied me down the hall to the ladies' ward, but was blocked by the Matron, whose body framed the doorway. She glared at Bill. "Sir, this is the ladies' ward. You are only allowed here to bring your wife's meals and toiletries." Bill ducked away, offering a little wave as I was led to my bed.

The Matron assisted me up onto Bed 9, a steel bed with a thin mattress covered in an even thinner yellow sheet. Then, a nurse in full uniform and cap, but without gloves, inserted a needle into my arm and attached a tube to an intravenous bag that she had hooked to a bent coat hanger fastened to the ceiling with a string. In horror, I saw this was not a rolling IV pole allowing mobility. I panicked. I was desperate for a toilet.

"I have to go to the bathroom, the water closet," I explained, my face contorted in fear that I might not make it. The nurse removed the IV from my arm and led me down a long hallway to the bathroom. There were three stalls, and each had a squat toilet sunk into the concrete floor. I groaned.

I was weak. There was nothing to grab to steady myself. I clung to my knees, hoping not to lose my balance. The diarrhoea flew from my body like a projectile.

I had a real mess going on. There was no toilet paper, just a bucket of water and a jug. I sloshed water as best I could to move the mess into the toilet. I poured water over my backside too.

I was wearing my street clothes and the water on the floor was above the level of my flip-flops. I squished all the way back to the ward and lay down upon the bed. The nurse hooked the IV back up, and I fell asleep.

The nurse took some blood in the morning. They were testing for Dengue, food poisoning and water-borne parasites. I advised I still had itchy skin and that a persistent chest cough had surfaced.

Food was not supplied at the hospital. Rice and curry and milk tea was brought to individual patients by family members referred to as 'by-standers'. Each night, the other patients' by-standers spread out red or blue bamboo mats or flattened cardboard on the concrete floor. In the night gloom of the darkened room, I tiptoed over these sleeping by-standers as I made my way to the toilet.

My bystander was kicked out, as he was male, but he was allowed to bring me ginger tea and fruit each day, along with some cheese and *parippu* crackers made from chickpea flour.

Co-patients peered at me. Timidly, I returned their gaze. They were friendly, despite us not having a common language. I'd shake my head and rub my stomach in response to the kind women who offered me some of their curry.

They tried adjusting the drip on my IV pole when they felt it was not flowing enough, they called the nurses when the IV pouch was empty, held the Band-Aids for the nurses with their unsterile hands, poured water into my mouth, stared at me at length from the end of my metal bed, and giggled at my visiting husband.

Each day, I improved and became more aware and curious about my surroundings and the people around me. There were about forty patients in the ward with beds for thirty people. I lay on my side on the narrow steel cot with no pillow and no blanket, watching them, my eyes louvred like slats like venetian blinds.

The daily ablutions performed by the women fascinated me. The women brushed their teeth using their forefinger as a toothbrush. Daily, they released their waist length black hair that had been confined to a bun at the nape of their necks and combed the tresses with a large toothy comb.

They looked at themselves in a tiny handheld mirror they each seemed to own, and then rubbed coconut oil into their hair before wrapping it back into a bun, smoothing away flyaway strands with oily hands. They rubbed white flour into their faces as a cosmetic. White flour or bleaching agents in skin lotions were a common beauty product for woman and children. White skin was valued.

Most of the women slept in their sari. Some of them did have a nightdress for sleeping, but each morning wrapped themselves in a bright sari swiftly, efficiently and effortlessly. I peeked, making mental notes as they wrapped, pinned and pleated.

After some days, a female physician, dressed in a red and gold sari, diagnosed my condition as acute gastroenteritis, and when I quizzed her about aetiology, she reported that she believed it was a food poisoning or the result of water-borne bacteria. There seemed no explanation for the skin itch or the cough.

She said I was discharged and advised that, as I was a foreigner, there would be a cost assessed to me. I fished out my cell phone from the pocket of my tunic and called my husband with the good news.

Once I was settled back into our house, Bill returned to the bustling, raucous Jaffna market to fetch some groceries. After he left, I needed to do something in private. I felt a need to honour the women who lay with me in the hospital beds— the women, who modestly dressed in front of me without a curtain to provide them privacy.

I shuffled into our bedroom and opened the tall brown wardrobe. From the wardrobe, I removed my peach sari from its plastic sheath and laid it out on a small plastic chair that stood beside our double bed, sheeted in white. I undressed and stood in my underwear.

I saw myself reflected in the mirror that hung from the door of the wardrobe. My body had leaned out from the days of not eating, vomiting and having 'loose motions'. I peered at my face in the mirror. *Is that me?* I asked myself. I looked unfamiliar, smaller, diminished and wan, lines on either side of my mouth curved like draws on a mountain in twilight.

I pulled open a small dresser drawer and extracted the beige cotton underskirt scalloped with beige lace at the bottom. I stepped into the underskirt, drew it up over my hips and tied the cotton strings firmly at my waist. I removed the round lid of the small red and black painted wooden box I had bought in Kandy from a

Laksala (a government-owned store for native handicrafts). From the small box, I extracted a bundle of diaper pins and smaller safety pins.

I removed one of the diaper pins from the bundle, opened it and placed it between my lips. I took the corner of the sari, right side of the fabric facing out and starting at my right hip, I wrapped the fabric across my belly and around my body, across my buttocks and safety pinned the fabric at my right hip. Next, I brought the remaining length of fabric around the back of my hips and in front of my navel.

I had learned to tie the sari by spying on my fellow patients at the hospital. Somehow, I felt a kinship with them. The beautiful garment was a symbol of our shared womanhood, our shared femininity. While dressing myself, I felt a sense of self-nurturing that I had never allowed myself.

I felt weak. I had just been discharged from the hospital. I gathered up my colourful skirts, unzipped the gauzy mosquito net that encased our bed, and crawled into the opening. I drew my folded skirt in with me and zipped the mosquito net closed.

I sat up in the bed with my legs straight out and smoothed the fabric out to my toes. I pulled the *pallu* forward, laying it across my concave belly. I lay upon the white pillow, still indented from the last day I had slept there. The pillow, familiar with my cranium, deeply cradled my head. I closed my eyes.

A prayer whispered across my lips. *Thank you for the gift of being sick. Thank you for allowing me to enter into relationship with other women who were sick. Thank you for allowing those women to teach me how to be stoic. Thank you for those who cared for me.* The words emitted from my brain were unspoken, silent and holy, sending out ripples of love to women everywhere.

When Bill returned, I was in sweet repose in my papaya-coloured sari. I dreamed of swirling silver and meshed golden threads dangling from elephant tusks and treetops with gold leaf borders, sequins glued to majestic purple fabric that sparkled in the azure sky. From puffy white clouds hung tassels of moonlight while brown hands tucked waves of love around me.

Tiny hands were pleating ribbons of blue water and between their full mouths they held tinkling silvery pins. I shifted. Bill backed out of the room and tiptoed away to the kitchen.

A month later, I still had not received a hospital bill. I asked one of the doctors I knew in Jaffna if he had any idea how long it might take to get the invoice. He became indignant. "We have free health care in this country. They cannot, and better not, charge you. You leave this to me."

"No, no, I am happy to pay," I protested. "I do not contribute to the taxes here."

"It doesn't matter, Wendy. Billing for health care would undermine our government system." I never did get a bill.

It was interesting having a patient perspective of Sri Lankan hospital care and to contrast it with hospital care in Canada. I had worked in a hospital long enough in Canada to know that the standards of cleanliness, regular equipment upgrades and state of the art beds were lovely, but perhaps not critical to health care.

The hospital in Jaffna was not pretty, but it was functional. They treated me well and now I was back at work, however, a persistent cough continued that seemed to keep me weak and tired and the tug to return home intensified.

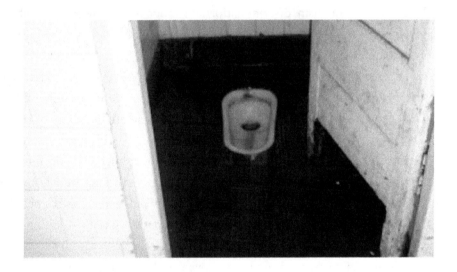

The bathroom at the hospital. Yup, I used this - many times

Chapter 31
A Trip to the Cage

I've never been to war, but I know the effects of war. War can never be a
solution because it creates greater problems than it solves.

Bill and I had both finished the book called *The Cage* by Gordon Weiss. We couldn't put it down. It is a book about the history of the war between the Sri Lankan Army (SLA) and the Liberation Tigers of Tamil Elam (LTTE). It is a disturbing account of racism, discrimination and struggles for power. The author paradoxically begins the book at the end of the Sri Lankan war with the killing of Prabhakaran, the LTTE leader.

The Cage is Nandikadal Lagoon in the northeast of Sri Lanka, where terrible things happened during the war. Weiss described how people were fleeing from the SLA. "Thousands of people streamed across the lagoon to the safety of army lines" (p. 211).

There were, "...apocalyptic scenes of children being dropped into the muddy water while their parents moved on, of mothers dying and their infants being scooped up, of an infant suckling on the breast of her dead mother, and of people being trampled underfoot in the stampede to escape the ghastly Cage inside which so many had already perished" (p. 212).

Since the end of the war, this region had been cordoned off by the Sri Lankan military, and nobody, neither Tamil nor Sinhala, was allowed into the area. However, we began to hear rumours that the Sinhalese people were being allowed in to see Prabakaran's camp and the killing fields. To better understand the context of the war, we made some inquiries and obtained the name of a young Sinhala man whose father had been killed in the Vanni and who had permission to go inside.

The Vanni is a triangular region between Jaffna, Mullaitivu and Kilinochchi and the region most affected by the final days of the war. Inside the Vanni is

Pathukuddiyiruppu, the site of Prabhakaran's personal bunker hideout and the Nandikadal Lagoon.

The night before the tour, Jo, Mary, Bill, Marcia, Anne and I took the bus down to Mullaitivo and stayed the night in a guesthouse with a murky swimming pool. The next morning, our tour guide arrived at the guesthouse in a white pickup to take us on the tour.

We pulled up to a site in a clearing where there was a monument announcing the location of the LTTE military museum. The rather meagre museum was filled with spent mortar casings, explosives, uniforms, rifles and some small boats used by the LTTE navy, including a half-finished torpedo boat. In addition, there were photographs, including a publicised photograph of the dead Prabakaran, a bullet through his forehead and photos of his children, also assassinated.

Next, our driver sped along the bumpy roads to Prabakaran's bunker. It was well hidden in the jungle with camouflage-coloured netting all around the perimeter. A set of narrow concrete steps led down to the small underground bunker painted blue throughout where there were living space, radio rooms and bedrooms. The grounds outside the bunker had large outdoor kitchens and a huge well where Sinhalese soldiers dressed in battle fatigue pants and khaki T-shirts were working.

All the Jaffna Family found the day sobering. As we drove home, we discussed what it must have been like for the Tamil people caught inside The Cage. That night, I was unable to sleep. I was too disturbed. Images and words filtered through my brain.

Three hundred thousand people had been trapped in the Cage. I saw the Dutch ship that had attempted to rescue people from the lagoon. I visualised the women rushing, children held high, wading out into the water in their bright saris, the water making the fabric cling to their legs like chains as they struggled towards the ship.

Then in my mind's eye, I saw the ship being ripped open with bullets and the people dunking under the water. There were pictures of dead women and children stranded by the morass of war. They floated in a slosh of red salt water.

I saw the images of bicycles piled high in a drought-filled dead terrain. Stacks of rusted dump trucks, school buses and bulldozers—all abandoned. Bombed houses, once family homes, now in ruin and full of holes. I saw the remnants of an old tent city where people were squeezed into the Vanni by the fighting.

The images were so real. I lay sweating under the mosquito net beside the slumbering Bill and Judge. I got up and quietly padded across our cement floor to the living room. In the dark, I switched on the computer and the glow illuminated the room. Trying to purge the terrible images, I started writing.

I think it was the piled mountain of bikes that made the people real to me. Thousands of red, rusty bicycles, now stripped of any rubber, piled up along a full mile of the dry, dusty road. Abandoned. Their riders dead or unable to claim the bikes back.

This pile of bicycles shook my equilibrium to its core. It depicted the mass of displacement, death and the waste of war. I wept as I imagined the final hours of the war.

Even though the war had been over for two years, its physical evidence was visible everywhere: bombed and shelled homes, abandoned homes, Sinhala soldiers at checkpoints, and people on the street with burns and missing limbs. Yet, I knew that the visible aspects of war were not the most damaging.

The real scars of war are the invisible ones, the ones carried inside the mind and stored in the memory. The emotional trauma that was being revealed to me was the real travesty of war.

Sadhika, one of my warm and generous colleagues, invited Bill and me to go for a drive with her and her husband, Mihir. We were excited to explore Jaffna with a couple we knew had remained in the area during the war. So, one Sunday, after mass, we headed out in their SUV towards the northern points of Jaffna, near the Tellipalai Hospital.

As Mihir drove along the beach front towards Point Pedro, he confirmed what we had already heard. "Much of the beach area was in the demilitarised zone and therefore, off limits. People owning land and housing in this area had their property expropriated by the army."

Sadhika turned her head to look at us in the back of the vehicle and explained, "During the height of the war, people fled without documents, and these documents were often destroyed during the war, making it difficult to provide proof of ownership to a sceptical government." We shook our heads in dismay.

Mihir then drove us into a shelled, overgrown neighbourhood. He stopped in front of a house, devoid of roofing tiles, windows and doors. "This was my house," he said tearfully.

"This is only the second time in twenty years I have been back here. The first time was right after the evacuation. I came back to see if some members of my family were still alive. Starving dogs were eating the corpses of my family and neighbours. I was horrified and I fled. I have not been back since, until today." He wept silently as Bill and I looked towards his destroyed home.

As we drove around the dusty, abandoned villages, Sadhika told us about the day the Indian Peace Keeping Force (IPKF) arrived in Jaffna. Initially, they had been sent to Sri Lanka as peacekeepers, but later, they started to provide food and medicine, and reputedly, arms to the LTTE. When the military agreed to a ceasefire, the LTTE did not. So, for three years, the Indian Army besieged Jaffna.

During one of these sieges, Sadhika, who worked as counsellor, ran towards the cupboard where confidential files were stored, gathered them up in her arms, and only then fled for her own safety amid the gunfire. These files contained evidence of people tortured for information by the Sri Lankan Army and who, in hope of restored mental health, had disclosed their torture.

Revelation of the identity of the people in these files would mean certain death or persecution. I did not need to teach my Sri Lankan colleagues about the protection and safekeeping of client files. They were experts at it.

Bill and I both felt somewhat fragile after visiting and hearing Sandhika and Mihir's stories. For the first time, we both sunk at the same time emotionally. It was sobering for us to think about these events for what they were, the deliberate murder of innocent people.

The war and the stories were bearing down upon me, weighing me down. I was drinking wine every night to cope.

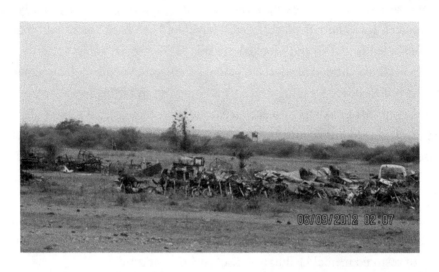

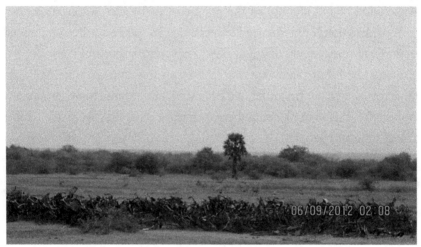

**Inside the Cage: The evidence left behind by civilians fleeing the war:
Mounds of bicycles and motorcycles**

Chapter 32
Learning from Torture and Trauma

Torture harms the tortured in different ways than it harms the torturer.

As the months passed by, I realised I was running out of time on the work front. For the better part of the year, and off the side of my desk, I developed a concept paper. The paper's premise was that Sri Lanka needed to provide a postgraduate diploma program in social work to fulfil the mandate of the Mental Health Policy of Sri Lanka.

This glossy policy called for a social worker to be in *every* Medical Officer Health (MOH) division by 2015. There were more than two hundred MOH divisions and very few social workers with actual degrees in social work in the country.

Stakeholders from the World Health Organisation (WHO), VSO and Sri Jayewardenepura University, along with two local and dedicated social workers, began meeting to address this shortage. At the same time, this committee was also addressing a necessary change at a structural level.

In Sri Lanka, as in most countries, the government is in control of the structures and infrastructures of the society. Without social work independence, it is very difficult for social workers to champion for the oppressed. Social workers cannot be 'puppets' of a government; they must be free to advocate for change and the breakdown of social and political structures that oppress.

They must be able to evolve as a profession without government interference. Thus, we needed to develop a 'fast track' method of graduating independent social workers from an independent university. This program was designed to ladder into a master's program in social work.

The University Grants Commission (UGC) accepted our proposal, and the Dean at Sri Jayewardenepura University was eager to offer the program. There was much to be done. The program needed approval from the Senate at the

University, curriculum needed to be developed, and a social work library for the program was to be established.

Textbooks were a rare commodity in Sri Lanka and with limited computer access or electronic library support, both students and instructors would require academic resource materials. I drafted an email to my social work colleagues in Kamloops. I pleaded for used, good condition social work textbooks.

Veteran social workers and new grads responded by culling their bookshelves and offering books for the cause. One of my professors from the bachelor's degree program, Trish Archibald, offered to be the 'collection depot'. She sorted the books, eliminated duplicates, fundraised for the shipping costs, boxed them up for the long journey, and posted the boxes to the VSO office in Colombo.

When they arrived, I cut back the packing tape and lifted the brown cardboard flaps of the crumpled boxes that had endured the voyage from Canada to Sri Lanka. Lovingly, I ran my hands over the worn covers of these old friends. I knew the words and work inside these books like the back of my hand.

These books were like teachers who imparted to me core social work knowledge, values and skills. Some were mentors who challenged my beliefs and assumptions. Others trained me in the art and science of social work. These books shaped my understanding of diversity and culture and furnished theory to guide my practice.

Tears slid down my cheeks. I was awash with gratitude that I was led to a profession that served me so well and one that allowed me to serve. These authors were guiding me now and I clung to their wisdom.

Now with these resources at my fingertips, I began writing curricula for the first semester. Marcia and Kamal, also both holding PhDs, agreed to write courses as well. Our goal was to have one full year of curriculum written to at least begin the program. We borrowed from social work course outlines from prestigious Canadian and UK universities to assist us.

At the same time, I worked with a group of people called the Trauma Team. The Trauma Team was established to support Tamil people tortured by the Sri Lankan government during the thirty-year civil war.

To assist in training the team, I had to know more about torture. As I had no prior knowledge of the motives of torturers, the psychology of torture, or the feelings of the tortured, it was important for me to research this most disturbing aspect of war.

I viewed websites and YouTube videos of tongues being cut off, people pushed off buildings, beheadings, waterboarding and electrical shock. I read academic research and journal articles on the subject. In the articles, researchers who had interviewed torture victims were able to identify the victim's worst fears. Interestingly, the type of torture applied was not as horrible as not knowing which torture would be used next and when the next torture was coming.

I told no one at that time of my research and my findings. When watching the film clips, I felt as though I was watching something illegal. This is how a person must feel when watching pornography and searching deeper and deeper for ever more disordered sex.

It was like a portal to hell sucking me into a vortex of visual and visceral horror. I returned to the clips more often than I should have, as though the images and atrocities were somehow addicting me to the horror. It began to feel like an obsession or an addiction.

These images had a profound impact on me. They began infecting my thinking and brought on disturbing dreams that sabotaged my sleep. I knew I needed to take these feelings to Jesus. Only he would understand me.

As I knelt in my tiny chapel on the beach one morning after a sleepless night, I gazed at the crucified Christ dangling on the cross. I considered the events at the time of His own death.

In the garden, just before he was tried and handed over to be crucified, Jesus himself must have experienced some of the same feelings the tortured men had described in the research I had studied. The literature described that the tortured experienced extreme agitation, anxiety and fear. The apostles who were with Jesus in the garden described that He suffered from the same emotions. In fact, He even begged his Father in Heaven to relieve him of his promise to die for the sins of mankind.

I considered His torture. To humiliate him, Roman soldiers stripped him of his clothing, spat upon him and mocked him by embedding a crown of thorns into his skull. He was whipped to near death and forced to carry a heavy cross through crowds that jeered at him.

His hands and feet were nailed with spikes to a cross. He was stabbed by a lance and given sour wine when he was thirsty. He was left to hang on a cross, the weight of his body tearing at the flesh around the nails in his hands and feet until he expired. Jesus knew all about torture, I realised. He understood the monstrosity of it.

I prayed for guidance. I tried to understand the absolute horror of being a victim of torture and the immense difficulty it must take to recover from these deliberate acts of human cruelty. This knowledge is critical for a therapist, as I had to understand the horrendous impact on the body, mind, emotion and spirit of a person who endures torture. A therapist must be able to bear witness and to elicit and hear the story, without causing vicarious trauma to self or furthering harm to the victim.

I had to be able to withstand the intensity of the clients' narratives. If a therapist is unable to 'handle' the pain and thus, is unable to hear that story, then the client is left bereft, without hope.

I began to feel different. It was as though I had somehow left behind the innocence created by the peace, privilege and security of Canada and had somehow joined the Tamil people in their struggle for rights and justice within their own country. I was undergoing some sort of internal change that left me feeling fragile and unprepared.

The Trauma Team also needed to understand the dynamics of torture and to prepare to engage more fully with the tortured. My counselling/training room was becoming a place of disclosure, revelation, pain and relief, not only for the therapists I was training, but also for my translator and myself. A large part of my training was modelling counselling skills, particularly group skills.

The therapists I was training were trying to run groups in the communities they served. These often-isolated communities had all experienced the effects of war, and many of them had also been impacted by the 2004 tsunami that shattered the villages in the Point Pedro area, killing many of the villagers and displacing thousands.

From February to June, I taught counselling skills to my students. They began using the skills when they took turns between being therapist and client during our twice a week group sessions. The team then took the skills into the villages and towns where the war affected lived.

Following an hour of therapy, we used the second hour for the students to discuss the curative factors evident in the session and to identify the skills used by the therapists that they had observed. They also had the opportunity to look at the effect of the skill on the client and to study the efficacy of each skill.

Students learned to watch for the group dynamic, analyse the sessions and look at the client's perceptions of events. I also taught them the importance of reflexive practice - the ability to see how the therapy, process and disclosures affect a therapist.

During this time, we became very close. I had been allowed to 'join' the group, which is a very critical part of group therapy as it is indicative of trust. One day, when it was Rahana's time to share, she told a story about her sister's death—she had been killed during the war. Her death left Rahana, a single woman, to raise her dead sister's children.

She described the heavy loss of her only sister, the burden of single parenting her niece and nephew and the financial hardships this commitment foisted upon her. The most serious impact and sacrifice for her was the loss of her own potential to be married.

After the group was finished for the day, Vasuki, who helped me as a translator during all the sessions, followed me to my office and closed the door behind her. We often discussed group afterwards as she filled me in on the relevant cultural aspects. That day, however, she sat down and when I looked up, her brown eyes were swimming in tears and her lip was trembling.

"I'm finding it very hard to be here and listen to the stories," she said, tears sliding down her face. "They are too similar to my own story," she explained between sobs, as she reached for a Kleenex that poked from the box on my desk. "Wendy, did you know that my sister was assassinated during the war?"

Her sister was Rajini Thiranagama, a medical doctor and a human rights activist, and her story became internationally known after the Canadian National Film Board filmed a documentary about her, called *No More Tears Sister: Anatomy of hope and betrayal.*

Rajini and Vasuki's other sister, Nirmila, were members of the Tamil Tigers (LTTE). In 1983, Rajini lobbied heavily for the release of Nirmila, who had been imprisoned in 1982 under the Sri Lankan Prevention of Terrorism Act. In 1989, Rajini became sympathetic to the cause of the LTTE, who began taking matters into their own hands by carrying out clandestine bombings and killings to bring about change.

Tamil Tigers were being injured in these skirmishes and needed medical attention. Unable to take their 'soldiers' to hospital for treatment, the Tiger leadership approached Rajini, who agreed to treat the injured. Under the cover of darkness, she provided medical attention to the wounded men and women. However, as the war deepened and politically motivated killings on both sides increased, often bringing injury and death to civilians, Rajini, an idealist, reconsidered her position and decided to 'quit' the Tigers.

She and some of her colleagues formed an association called University Teachers for Human Rights. Rajini began collecting evidence to support human rights violations by the LTTE and the Indian Peace Keeping Force (IPKF) that had wreaked havoc in Jaffna from 1987 to 1989. The gathered evidence of human rights abuses and war crimes was compiled into a book called *The Broken Palmyra*.

On 21 September 1989, a few weeks following the release of *The Broken Palmyra*, Rajini was shot and killed while riding her bicycle home from work at the medical faculty in Thirunelvely, Jaffna. The gunman was never found. It is believed by many that she was assassinated by the LTTE for having criticised them.

The day Vasuki shared this story with me, it had been a particularly challenging group session. People untrained to hear the tragic stories of others' lives can have a deep emotional reaction to the stories, especially when the story resonates with something they have experienced. Vasuki held her emotions in check during the group session, but in the privacy of my office, she broke down.

I normalised her feelings and supported her in knowing that sharing was an important part of the work. Her sharing of the story bonded me to her. She was a rare gift to me and to our group of therapists.

The impact of the stories was becoming difficult for me as well. I was a professional therapist and trained to bear witness to the painful stories of others, but this does not always prevent even an experienced therapist, like me, from having a story cross an emotional boundary. A story told in the group rocked me, too.

Narum had a brilliant smile and his self-deprecating comments often made us laugh. He was liked and respected by the group. He spoke a bit of English and the telling of his story was a mixture of both Tamil and English. He spoke slowly, thoughtfully, providing rich detail of a night that occurred during the war.

He was fifteen years of age, and his father had just died of cancer. Grief-stricken, his mother had sunk into depression, rarely leaving her bed. Narum became the caregiver to his mother and his two younger siblings.

Three months after his father's funeral, Sinhala soldiers entered Jaffna, and an evacuation order was issued for all people to move to Chavakacheri, a small town to the south.

That night, Narum bundled rice, flour and other foodstuffs into sacks. He tied pots and pans, fuel and clothing to his bike and stuffed knapsacks and other bags with utensils and toiletries. He gathered his mother from her bed, gave her dark clothes to wear, dressed his sister and brother in black and in the dark of night, they ran to his loaded bicycle.

It was a common sight in Sri Lanka for whole families to be doubled on a bicycle, with the man of the family navigating the load; the wife on the centre bar of the bike, a child bundled in her arms, a small child perched on the handlebars, another child on a board behind the seat or standing on the back axles as the father pushed against the pedals.

However, that night, amidst the bomb blasts, Narum was unable to get the bike going with the load of belongings and his family members. Despite several attempts to achieve balance and momentum, the bike was too heavy. Each time, the family and the belongings tumbled into the dust.

The mortar fire seemed closer and in desperation to leave, he stashed the large bag of rice in the house and planned to cycle back for it in the morning, once his family was safe with relatives in Chavakacheri. With the lightened load, Narum pushed the bike to a large chunk of cement that stood in a neighbour's abandoned yard, and his family clambered aboard. Once steady, he was able to push the bike forward with his left foot and with that momentum, veered down the dark, dirt road to Chavakacheri.

They joined a long line of other refugees fleeing Jaffna, each family laden with necessities taken from their homes, each person bewildered and frightened as they walked, pedalled or rode their motorcycle under the moonlight and flashes from nearby bombings and machine gun fire.

Due to the darkness, the potholes he could not see over his towering load, and the crowding from the other refugees, Narum fell three times, each time dumping his family onto the dark soil.

At one point, his little brother chose to walk to lighten the load and in the confusion along the way, went missing. Fear gripped them all, but all the family could do was continue to ride, hoping that the little boy was in the caravan of refugees. Narum prayed for the safety of his brother and railed at his father as he rode along. *Why did you leave us, Papa? We need you. I am too young to be responsible for the family.*

Eyes wet with tears, Narum said, "Somewhere near morning as we neared Chavakacheri, my little brother surfaced. I thought I had lost him too. I was so happy to see him." Sniffling could be heard in the room as he continued his story,

"We travelled to the home of my aunt and uncle. I deposited my family with them, then I advised my relatives that I was returning for the rice I had left behind. I told them I hoped to be back by dinnertime."

As the hot sun cast coral and reds at sunrise, Narum snuck back towards Jaffna on his bike. Littering the road were abandoned clothing and bags, evidence that fleeing families realised the importance of getting to safety superseded their belongings arriving safely. Narum darted in and out of the trees and shrubs when vehicles passed. When the road was clear, despite his fatigue, he cycled furiously towards the rice and sustenance it represented.

When he arrived home, the place was deserted and looked unharmed. He breathed a sigh of relief and propping his bike up against the fence, he carefully crossed the garden. The house door was wide open. He told us,

"The house had been ransacked, but there was nobody there. I crept to the closet where I had stashed the large bag of rice. I flung open the doors. The rice was gone! I thought I must be mistaken."

"I tore the house apart, looking in each cupboard, under beds, in closets, the bathroom. I looked everywhere, but it was gone. It must have been plundered by the Sinhala soldiers on their rampage through the city."

Realising he had returned in vain, Narum sank to his knees, placing his face upon the floor. He sobbed piteously, his body wracked with the pain at losing his father and, essentially, his mother, the loss of the normality of life, his interrupted education and the burden of responsibility now foisted upon him. He raged at his father for dying, his mother for avoiding responsibility with depression, and at his siblings for being young and useless.

Narum's rage spent itself, transforming to deep fatigue. He crawled to his bed and pulling the thin sheet about him, he fell into a deep sleep despite the distant mortar fire. As dusk approached and the mosquitos began chewing on his foot that stuck out from beneath the sheet, he arose, looked around one more time and slipped out of his home, closing the door behind him.

He mounted his bike and rode back to Chavakacheri. The dark closed around him as he cycled, fear chasing him.

Narum told his story with eloquence and grace. He sniffed and wiped his nose on the back of his hand. The group had been taught the value of therapeutic silence. It is in the silence of the waiting that the client often presents the dynamic of the situation. We all waited in silence. Finally, Narum spoke. "Something happened to me that night," he stated, his eyes luminous and fragile.

The silence was deafening. We allowed Narum the time and space to put his finger on the totality and essence of his story. "I lost my childhood," he finally whispered. "That night, I became a man."

We all wept. I was deeply affected. His story made the war even more real to me. I remembered the stack of bicycles I had seen at Mullativo. They represented families like Narum's. Reflexive practice was required for me to work through my own feelings. Being a mother myself, I wanted to protect that fifteen-year-old boy from having to shoulder such a heavy load.

I felt angry with his mother for not being more functional for her children. I couldn't help but think how helpless I might be in that circumstance with my five children. My anger passed as empathy deepened for children with depressed parents and as I realized the disabling effects of depression on parents.

The trauma of the therapists I was training undermined any confidence I had in my own ability to help. Any skills I believed I had seemed to vanish. I felt I had nothing to offer. I was a clinician from Canada. My practice involved, for the most part, working with patients with mental illness, persons who had suffered sexual abuse as children and couples struggling with marital issues.

At the chapel, I knelt. I looked at the represented Jesus on the cross and asked, "Lord, what do I have to offer people suffering from torture, killings, death, refugee camps and displacement? You brought me here unprepared," I accused Him. "Where do I go from here?"

Intuitively and silently, He responded to my fears and my plea for assistance. It became clear to me that I had to seek supervision. In my research, I had come across the work of Dr Daya Somasundaram, and his journal article entitled, "Collective Trauma in Northern Sri Lanka: a qualitative psychosocial-ecological study" and his book, *Scarred Minds*.

Dr Somasundaram was a psychiatrist and researcher, and he had been a major contributor to understanding the psychosocial effects of war on the people of northern Sri Lanka.

In 2016, as a co-author of *The Broken Palmyra*, and after Rajini was assassinated, he fled his home in Sri Lanka at the start of the 'final' war and sought refugee status in Australia. There, he became an associate professor at the University of Adelaide.

He returned to his home in Sri Lanka under the Scholar Rescue Fund, a fund used to return the intelligentsia back to the northern part of the island. As a founding member, he maintained a close tie to Shanthiham, where I was working. He agreed to meet with me and invited me to his home to hear my concerns and to provide direction.

The day of the appointment, I hopped on my scooter and headed out to Uduvil, the small village where he lived. It was very near to the place where Rajini had been murdered. He greeted me with a handshake as I entered his gate.

His blue plaid sarong was faded from multiple washings and drying in the hot sun. He wore a threadbare and yellowed T-shirt. His beard was stubble. His feet bare and dusty. He padded across the hard-packed earth in his yard towards two green plastic lawn chairs that stood facing one another under a mango tree. I followed. I had not met him before and was surprized by his lack of formality.

We sat on the chairs, sheltered from the hot afternoon sun. I began to tell him a bit about my professional background and that I was feeling overwhelmed by the stories; that I felt I had nothing to offer to the therapists. I told him that the Trauma Team knew more than I did in terms of how to counsel people affected by the war.

He listened, and at times, there were awkward silences. Then, he began to speak, measuring his words.

"Safety is the real issue," he advised me. "During the war, people learned they could not trust their neighbours and sometimes even their family members. Security forces on every corner was a form of intimidation, and the people felt unsafe. Jaffna is not an ideal clinical setting."

He advised me not to rely on the western approaches to therapy, but to use narrative exposure and storytelling to bring forward traumatic experiences. He explained, "Culturally, Tamil people use stories to bring meaning to their personal situations."

He encouraged me to ask about the stories that contributed to the family lore, the stories that accompanied their experiences during the war and the stories of survival.

He also encouraged the use of drawing and painting as a way of eliciting stories, rather than the western 'hot seat' approach. What he was saying made sense, although, I was not sure how *not* to rely on my western education and my western practice experience. He suggested trauma literature that focussed on indigenous cultures.

"Wendy, there is no right or wrong, no yes or no, there are just influences. Move away from the western model towards more indigenous approaches," he urged. He also suggested using relaxation, breathing, meditation and yoga as forms of therapy. He encouraged me to assist therapists to be flexible in treatment approaches and for them to focus on all domains: the social, the educational, their livelihood, the emotional and the spiritual.

He understood the difficulty in hearing the tragic and horrible stories. He encouraged me to seek supervision as often as necessary and to use peer support. He cautioned me, "Wendy, you need time and space to process what you hear. Don't overschedule yourself."

He provided me his email address to facilitate ongoing supervision. Leaving his yard and driving away into the heat on my scooter, I wept as I bumped along. I had felt so inadequate. But now, I had additional and even better tools that I could begin to apply in my practice.

That night, I thought about how to use narrative and visual arts. I had read about a timeline used in clinical practice for children traumatised in war. A string about three feet long is placed along the ground, and the child is given a few rocks and some plastic flowers.

One end of the string represents their birth, the other the present time. On their timelines, they are to place a flower for every good thing and a rock for every bad thing that happened, in the order they happened. Once the rocks and flowers are in place, the child can share the stories of what they represented.

I decided to use this technique as a starting point. The next morning, I went to the local shop and purchased bunches of plastic flowers. As Jaffna is built on sand, I used wadded paper packed into balls to represent rocks. I drew out timelines on large sheets of paper for each of my team members.

During our session, the group began to develop their timelines. Thoughtfully, they placed their flowers and rocks. It was shocking to see how few flowers there were on some timelines and how many rocks marked their lives.

The visual aid of the timelines allowed the stories to flow. My team of therapists felt safe, and they felt heard. New skills were introduced, and new skills were applied. Each week, the therapists took their new skills to the field and applied them to their own clients. Each week, they came back to the classroom and received coaching and supervision from me and peer support from their colleagues.

Dr Somasundaram's wisdom and the application of his cultural approach not only helped my team turn a corner personally and emotionally, but also professionally. I often sat in wonder after each session, feeling awash with humility after witnessing the stories that left these people so broken, so scarred, yet they continued, each day, to pick themselves up.

They embodied resilience. They continued to find joy and to give of themselves to their colleagues and their families. It was an honour and privilege to help share that burden. I felt my own resilience building as well. My work began to feel productive and curative and more importantly, I felt I was protected from doing further harm.

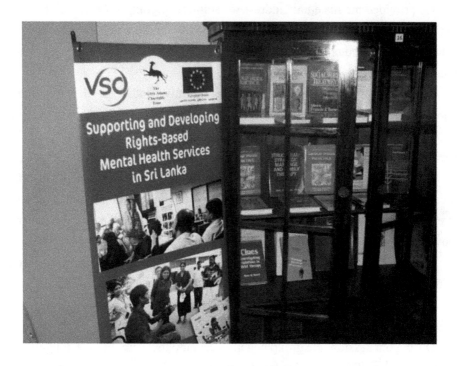

Social Work textbooks donated from Canadian and UK Social workers to build a library for a School of Social Work at Sri Jayewardenepura University in Colombo

Chapter 33
Goodbye to Sri Lanka

There really is no need to say goodbye as it takes merely a thought of you
to be there again.

On 28 November 2012, the last 2012 grandchild was born! It cheered us up. Shelley had promised not to deliver until we got home, but Colten, her baby son, had other ideas. He weighed 6 lbs 9 oz despite being three weeks early. Colten is Bill's first biological grandchild, and he was emotional, weeping at every photo that sped over the Internet. We knew we would be home soon to hold him and the other grandchildren we had not yet met.

My VSO contract was to expire the end of December 2012. However, VSO had requested that I extend my contract until March 2013. To everyone's surprise, the VSO mental health program was leaving Sri Lanka.

The World Bank had upgraded Sri Lanka from an underdeveloped country to a middle-income country, and as a result, the VSO head office decided to move their resources elsewhere. I was offered a work extension to assist with the closing of the program here.

I wanted to stay in Sri Lanka, but I desperately wanted to go home too. I was ambivalent, torn between my work and my family.

Instead of deciding, I ran to my little chapel. It was my last visit to my tiny sanctuary on the edge of the lagoon. The statue of Blessed Vaz continued to stand in the mud. He had protected the chapel where I had always received solace and direction over the past year.

I knelt again and poured my heart out. "You brought me here, Jesus, knowing full well that I have responsibilities at home. Now I have all these new grandchildren you have given me that I haven't even seen yet. But VSO wants me to stay longer, and you know I want to stay and close out the program. You need to make the decision because I can't.

I felt I had been heard. I declined the extension and gave my official notice to VSO. My last working day in Sri Lanka would be 14 December 2012. This date afforded sufficient time to close our home in Jaffna and say goodbye to our VSO colleagues scattered about the country. It also gave us time to make travel arrangements for Judge, Bill and me to be home for Christmas.

Our adventure in Sri Lanka was like a dream come true and provided something much more than mere travel. As tourists, Bill and I had travelled to many countries and had peered in at the people in a fishbowl. This time, we were residents, floundering about *within* the fishbowl. This unique experience plunged us into unfamiliar waters of culture, difference, sameness and language.

Within the fishbowl, it was challenging to navigate the daunting, jumbled, disordered and colourful marketplaces just to find the essentials of life. It was challenging to adjust to the pace, timing and lack of urgency in a collective culture, and it was difficult for me to balance ethnocentrism with capacity building in the workplace.

It was challenging to stay alive as we navigated the muddy, bumpy roads and rabid traffic. As one colleague joked, "Only convicted murders were allowed to apply as bus drivers."

Now we wanted to be out of the fishbowl. This desire crept up when we least suspected, catching us at vulnerable moments and leaving us awash with loneliness, a feeling of futility about my work, and a sense of entrapment. Inside the fishbowl, we felt isolated by colour, language and custom, and so we stared, our noses pressed against the glass, looking towards home.

We were always free to come home, but at times, it didn't feel as if we had that freedom of choice. We had undertaken a commitment to ourselves, to VSO, to the people of Sri Lanka, for the profession of social work, for human rights, for the mentally ill, and for peace. Yet, at times, it was hard to recall the values that had shaped our decision.

The two years away from home magnified into what seemed a much longer time. Now writing this, eleven years later, the time spent there has shrunk to what seems like mere months.

The weekend before coming home, steeped in nostalgia and wistfulness, we made a tour of our old haunts in Colombo. I sipped deep red wine on the lanterned patio of the Banana Leaf restaurant. We lounged on the pool deck of Cinnamon Grand Hotel savouring our last swim and the golden rays of the Sri Lankan sun.

We walked down Duplication Road and entered our gem shop. We shook hands, saying goodbye to Shaf, our jewellery maker. We met VSO friends for coffee at the Barefoot Restaurant, where large, colourful koi swam in a sun-dappled pond and the sun shone onto the open patio. I purchased a few knick-knacks for home, and then we headed to Padmini's for our final night in Sri Lanka.

In the past when we had stayed at Padmini's guesthouse, she had often sat with us over our breakfast, educating us on the culture and lifestyle of Sri Lanka in a friendly, but business-like manner. This time was different. Padmini swept into the living room, her bright caftan moving about her slippered feet. She carried whiskey glasses and sat them on the teak table.

"I want to have a glass of whiskey with you to say goodbye," she declared, moving to a side cupboard. Padmini was a grand woman, a remnant of colonialism and yet, an intellect and a shrewd businesswoman who was still evolving to keep pace with a modernising Sri Lanka.

She opened the dark wooden cupboard and selecting a twenty-six-ounce bottle of Canadian Club, she poured the amber liquid into the waiting crystal glass that stood before me. Then, she drained the amber liquid into her own glass. She secured the cap on the bottle and returned the bottle to its resting place in the cabinet and closed the door. She poured water into a crystal glass for Bill.

With grace and charm, she settled herself into her brocade armchair and bent her bejewelled fingers around the crystal glass. Warmly, she looked at the both of us. "Bon voyage," she said in perfect French. I raised my whiskey and Bill raised his water glass.

The crystal tinkled. A perfect goodbye. Padmini had been our first Sri Lankan host and now, our final host. We had gone full circle.

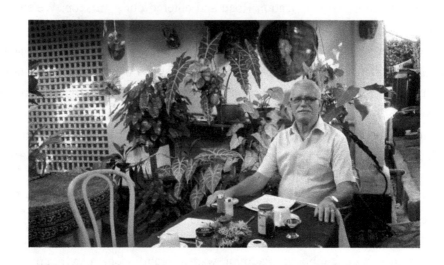

Our last breakfast in Padmini's garden patio in Colombo

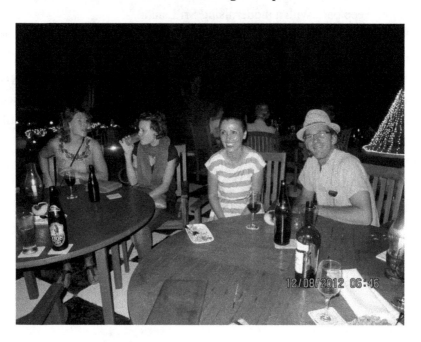

One of our final gatherings at Galle Face Green Hotel in Colombo with other VSO volunteers

Part Four
Re-Entry into Canada

Chapter 34
Back on the Farm

Travelling makes you see the world in technicolor and being home is like seeing in black and white.

We left Sri Lanka on 12 December and arrived back in Canada on 12 December 2012. We flew into time and were in the air a gruelling twenty-two hours! So was our poor kitty, Judge. She had been contained in a crate in the cargo hold during the flight.

As we had final meetings in Colombo before departing, Judge had to be kennelled in a veterinarian's office for five days prior to the long flight. Once we landed in Vancouver, we hustled to the car rental, secured a van and then sped to the cargo depot.

She was shivering, crying and hungry. We had lined her crate with a pet mattress pad designed to soak up urine discharged during the flight. It was surprisingly clean and dry. The can of cat food we had taped to her crate was still there, untouched.

Her non-spill water dish was empty. Grains of rice clinging to the mattress pad indicated some compassionate baggage handler had attempted to feed her.

After devouring her wet food, she was caged another four hours as we drove along the Coquihalla Highway to our home in Kamloops. It was December, but like the Red Sea parting for the Israelites, the winter weather parted for us, allowing us to drive home on bare and dry, summer-like roads. Were we fleeing Sri Lanka or being welcomed to the promised land?

Perhaps both and neither, but we knew we couldn't be in two places at the same time. It seemed we were being guided home as within hours of returning home, the clouds groaned under their stored weight and dumped their white loads. Over sixty centimetres of snow blanketed the ground over the next couple of days, reminding us that we were again in Canada, the land of ice and snow.

Our family was as anxious to see us as we were to see them. My mother prepared a delicious dinner for our arrival with our favourite foods and a houseful of our wonderful family greeted us: children, grandchildren, brothers, sisters, nieces and nephews, about thirty-seven loved ones in all.

Joyfully, we exchanged stories. We had missed so much over the two years we had been away. The kids had all grown a foot taller and the adults a bit older.

As our house was still rented until April, we moved into our ski condo for four months. Judge lived in front of the crackling wood fireplace, and Bill and I skied, read and entertained our family and friends. Finally, in April, we moved back into our home and slipped back into our lives here, as if never away.

A curtain was pulled over our life in Sri Lanka and we were left pinching ourselves, trying to remember we had lived there for two entire years. It felt so strange.

What was even more strange is that it seemed nobody was curious about what had taken place for us in Sri Lanka. Very few people asked me about my work, and if they did, accepted a superficial answer.

Whenever I attempted to provide a bit more detail, my listeners' eyes glazed over and before long, the conversation turned towards current events or events of their life in the past two years. Now I believe that despite good intentions, the experience is beyond most people's understanding, as they cannot feel the emotional impact it had upon us.

CUSO has long recognised the phenomenon that occurs when volunteers return home. As part of the holistic volunteer process, they have built into the process a re-integration weekend. So, a few months after we returned home, we flew to Ottawa again.

Canadian and American volunteers who had been deployed to Jamaica, Africa, Nigeria and other countries met in the CUSO/VSO office to discuss their experiences in a guided fashion. It turned out that all of us had the same sense of feeling like 'we have never been away' and 'nobody understands what we went through' and 'people just glaze over when we speak about our experience.'

Also, all volunteers had stories that impacted them. We felt heard by each other. One of the guided exercises was for us to draw a picture depicting an event or an incident that impacted us the most. In red felt pen, I drew a picture of the night when Narum fled Jaffna in the middle of the night, carrying his family on one bicycle.

I drew in the beautiful palmyra trees and the stars and the moon that contrasted with the bombs that exploded around him. I drew the goods heaped upon the bike as he and his family began their exodus. As I drew, I felt my lips trembling.

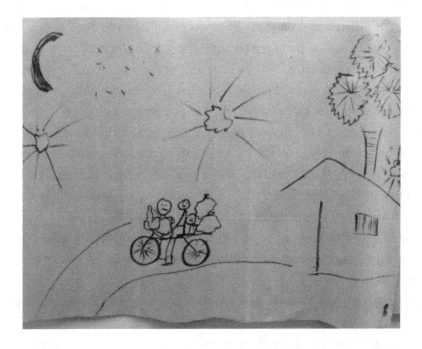

When it was my turn to share my story, I wept. I realised the impact of Narum's story on me, and the cumulative effect of all the stories told by the volunteers, the collective experience of the people of Jaffna, and the stress of our re-integration back to Canada. I sat down, hiding my face in a tissue. Narum's story was his rite of passage from childhood to manhood.

As I wept, I realised why Narum's story resonated so deeply for me. I had undergone my own rite of passage. I had been transformed by the separation, the experience and the return home. I felt less cowardly, more resilient and more certain I was prepared for whatever challenges lay ahead in my life.

Flying home from Ottawa, I stared out the window of the airplane that was flying through a light fog. I reflected on the experience and asked myself tough questions for which I had no answers. *Had I made a difference? Did I bring about any real change? Was the work sustainable?*

I shifted in my seat as the plane bumped along. I closed my eyes. *Will anything be different because of my work?*

My brain scoffed, "Nope." As the program closed after we left the country, no follow-up was done. From a measurable standpoint, there was not a scrap of evidence that any difference was made. Development, from that standpoint, was a failure.

However, my soul replied to the questions with a different answer. "Yes, you did make a difference. You made an impact on those you taught. You valued them as people and as people who had suffered. You shared with them your knowledge and experience."

If nothing else, to those I taught, I planted seeds of new skills, new ways of looking and doing things. I planted seeds of respect for each other regardless of colour, race or caste. I bridged cultures by being open and honest about the good, bad and ugly in my own culture. I gave of myself and that, surely, must matter.

Guastello (1997) described the 'butterfly effect' as, "a small change…at the right place in time" that "can produce a large effect elsewhere in the system" (p. 345). I hoped that I was in the right place at the right time.

I hold onto this scrap of hope, otherwise a sense of futility descends upon me. I sought constant reassurance from God that all my efforts were not futile. He gave me comfort.

A full five years after we had returned home, a restlessness and nagging feeling took over again. Bill explained it by reminding me of the famous World War I song, "How you gonna keep them down on the farm after they've seen Paree?" We had been to Paree, and now we had to live back 'on the farm'.

I began to understand that discontent is the human condition. We begin to long for something and when the longing turns into a burning desire, the person is compelled to take action to fulfil that desire at all costs. Yet, when that dream is fulfilled, there is but a brief period of time when desire is satisfied, quiet and still.

Then, the stirring of discontent begins again, invading the soul. The spirit becomes restless again for the next thing to do. We set a new goal not for the mere sake of accomplishment, but more as a quest born out of curiosity. It is an uncomfortable disquiet.

It was difficult, at first, to discern what the disquiet was telling me. It began as a whisper, a vague disturbance, veiled and unformed, but distinct, like a gnawing or an anxiety without form or substance. It began to take shape as a desire to do something and dusted into an intense storm. I realised I needed to write our story.

The events of our life transpired because of finding that newspaper article about CUSO. These events needed to be documented to provide some immortality and memory to the events. Without their record, like pencil sketches fading with time, the memories would blur, become indiscernible and finally, gone. The only evidence being a smudge, like an oily fingerprint upon paper.

The adventures, larks, troubles and trials of our life in Sri Lanka seemed easy to pen at the time as they flowed from the abundance of experiences. What is much harder to get at, to articulate, to perceive, never mind share, is how those experiences shaped us and what makes it so hard for us to settle down here, on the farm.

However, with time, the insights as to the meaning and purpose of our journey emerged. It has been nearly fifteen years since we began the application process, thirteen years since we first stepped into Ceylon, and eleven years since we came home. Some of the rich detail eludes me when I re-imagine a scene, hoping to describe it in the way it justly deserves.

By writing these memoirs, I turned and dug into each story like sod, to examine their impact upon me. By giving the stories form, I can continue my reflexive practice of the events that occurred in Sri Lanka. It can be an ongoing, lifelong process.

Bill and I integrated some of the language and culture into our everyday life. These remnants conjure up memories of our time there. My favourite is when someone asks me my name. My memory whispers, 'Mage Nama Wendy' before I respond in English, "My name is Wendy."

Bill uses a hand gesture. He holds up his arm straight in front of his body with his fingers held tightly together. Then, he flaps his wrist up and down, while he says, "Come, come." This hand gesture is used by both the Sinhala and the Tamil to wave you forward into a room or an office.

Bill still waves people into our home with this gesture and uses it when he wants to show me something. These quirks acquired in Sri Lanka now seem indelible and intrinsic, like a genetic archetype, a remnant from our experience.

The storm to write converged with another event. In 2017, Bill was diagnosed with Alzheimer's Disease. Receiving the diagnosis made me put to bed the notion that another CUSO adventure was possible. I resigned myself to live vicariously through our own lived experience and through the reconstruction of the stories that lay stored but were quickly decaying. After Bill's diagnosis, I finally drew back the curtain and resurrected the memories.

To start the process, I had to tackle the three Tetra packs of photos and a plastic storage bin of memorabilia that we had accumulated from our trip. I used these and the blogs I had written to help resurface memories.

I soon realised that there was an aspect of working overseas that we had not foreseen. Even though I was working full time, and harder than I had ever worked, in cultures and languages unknown, there was a carefree sense of freedom, a lack of responsibility. I think all the VSO volunteers felt it.

There were no family to visit, no hobbies to tend to. There were no obligations, save those of the critical work for which we had volunteered. In a sense, we were freer than we had been at home.

There was, and continues to be, a curative factor that comes from our work in Sri Lanka. I had never moved away from my home community before. I had always enjoyed the safety of a large family and a bank of friends from childhood, high school and university. But I had always felt as though something was missing from my development.

By going to Sri Lanka, I was forced to individuate. It was a rite of passage for me; I felt myself maturing and expanding. I was forced to make new friends and develop a network of people. Our 'Jaffna Family' met all the criteria of love, connection, a sense of belonging and acceptance that a family should supply.

It was curative for me in other ways. As I had received my PhD only a couple of years before moving to Sri Lanka, I didn't have an opportunity to apply all my knowledge in my clinical practice or in further research. I had felt a bit of a fraud. Working in Sri Lanka was a double-edged sword; I had the credentials but did not yet know how to wield the learning. It was humbling.

The more I worked in my profession in Sri Lanka, the more I realised that the principles of self-determination, unconditional personal regard and respect for diversity were transferable across culture, country and race. I began to fence with my sword. I did have something to offer others, and in return, they had something to offer me. It was a reciprocal relationship and in that, it cured me of my imposter syndrome, of not being good enough.

Social work is a blend of art and science. I began to feel that I had integrated my education with my personality, my creativity and the dynamic of my relationships with people to achieve the artistic aspect. This blend seemed valued by others, and I began to value myself as my potentials were being unveiled.

Today, as I sit looking out at the hush that comes with the first snowfall of this winter of 2022, we are again facing another long cold winter. But now, the memories are documented, standing in the wings to comfort Bill and I whenever we need refreshment, or we yearn for quest and freedom. They await us, ready to explode upon our senses when we need to re-experience the pungency of ripe papaya and the noise and beauty and splendour of an exotic land.

They are suspended, waiting for us to lick our fingers and turn a page where we can again feel the vibrancy of change, where we stand on a mountain witnessing a vista of shimmering colours and marvels that leave us shaking in awe.

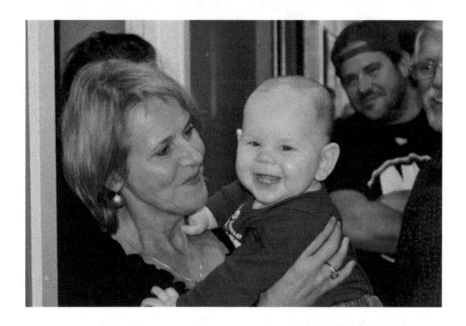

December 2012: Meeting grandson, Michael, for the first time

Epilogue

A passage from the book, *The Black Robe* by Wilkie Collins, resonated with me. In the story, Bernard Winterfield, a character in the novel, wryly records in his diary:

"It strikes me that I am falling into a bad habit of writing too much about myself. The custom of keeping a journal certainly has this drawback...it encourages egotism. Well, the remedy is easy. From this date, I will lock up my book...only to open it again when some event has happened which has a claim to be recorded for its own sake. As for myself and my feelings, they have made their last appearance in these pages."

Like Mr Winterfield, my experience in Sri Lanka had a claim to be recorded for its own sake. Already, I have tarried. By recording these events, I now possess a storage vessel of stories sealed between the covers of a book and thus, it prevents my rapidly receding memories from totally abandoning me.

The memories and my feelings about those memories are locked onto pages where they can no longer slip away. They are indelible. And soon, I shall put aside both my ego and my journal, and like Mr Winterfield, make my last appearance.

The stories leave a legacy for my children and grandchildren about what their mother and grandmother was up to when she disappeared to Sri Lanka.

As well, and perhaps more importantly, the story asks questions about life. Can the reader hold strong spiritual beliefs that guide and support them, yet have respect for the religious beliefs and values of those with whom they interact? I was a social worker, not a missionary. My faith was internal and private but critical support for me to do my work.

Can the reader do volunteer work as well? Can the reader find meaning and purpose in life by seeking and grasping opportunity? The legacy to the readers of *Indelible* is that meaning and purpose in life and opportunities exist around every corner.

Chamali and I have telephoned once or twice since I left Sri Lanka. I wrote to her at Christmas for two years but did not receive any letter back. I did not know if I had the correct address anymore.

Three years ago, I was able to contact her sister on Facebook, and she informed me that my beloved Chamali did get my notes. Chamali now has her own Facebook and posts pictures of her two children and writes to me from time to time.

Marjorie and her husband, Richard, became fast friends of ours in Sri Lanka, and since that time, they have travelled to Canada to see us. We spent three weeks bombing about in a rickety motorhome across BC, sipping wine and hiking. In turn, we spent a week in England with them, and then together, we motored our way across the Chunnel to France, where we enjoyed time in their medieval second home.

We toured together in Spain's Costa Brava and have swum in the Mediterranean. We swam and cycled in Mexico and cycled from Passau, Germany to Budapest, Hungary. We have cycled mountainous climbs along the Amalfi Coast in Southern Italy.

Gerd and Maria continued in Sri Lanka after we left. Other than an occasional email, Bill and I hadn't heard much from them. However, in 2015, when I was teaching International Social Work, a fourth-year Bachelor of Social Work course at Thompson Rivers University, I contacted Gerd and asked him to consider being a guest speaker via Skype for my students.

Gerd had continued working for the UN World Food Program and at that time was working in Ukraine, delivering food assistance to the vulnerable regions of Donetsk and Luhansk. He agreed. He described for my keen students how food was provided by the NGO and the situation on the ground in Ukraine at that time. It was wonderful to speak to him and to introduce him to my students.

In the fall of 2018, Gerd contacted us. He asked if we knew anyone in Canada who might support his brother, Olsi, to leave Albania. Albania, a country released from communism in 1990, left young men like Olsi without suitable employment, despite a university education.

After brief consideration, Bill and I agreed to have Olsi live with us. He arrived in April 2019, pursued additional education and now has sustainable employment. Like his brother, he was wonderful to be around. We have regular contact.

Jo Coombs, a member of our Jaffna Family met Beth Gee, another VSO occupational therapist living and working in Colombo. They became fast friends, and then more than that. Their relationship culminated with their wedding in September 2017. They reside in Brighton, England with their little dog, Muffin.

Kamal and I keep in touch in our Christmas letters. As we both love writing, we sometimes share our writing work with each other. She lives in London and is working as a psychologist.

Marcia Brophy was my closest VSO partner and friend. We shared an office, and we shared a home. Marcia continued with NGO work after Sri Lanka. She and Mischi, who still lives in Puttalam, continue their relationship. I remain connected to them in my heart.

Mary Cuttle and Anne Murray continue in our hearts as well. Bill and I are often amused at their Facebook posts from around the world. We only need to find the time, money or excuse to reconnect, and most of us will find each other again. Anne is currently working in Myanmar.

Shaun Humphries and Trina Cobbledick were the only other Canadian volunteers in Sri Lanka. It was nice to hear familiar accents and to dive with them in the Maldives. They now live in Malaysia.

There were other VSOs working in Sri Lanka at the time. While they were all wonderful colleagues, our lives and work crossed infrequently. However, when we all came together at the same time, whether in Colombo or elsewhere, we all enjoyed each other so much.

We felt lucky to be so like-minded. Again, it felt like serendipity. Many of us did meet for a reunion in England in 2017. We continue to remain connected by a Facebook group entitled, *And Back to VSO Volunteers Sri Lanka*.

Mark and Sewwandi continue their life in Leeds and we have seen them on a couple of occasions. One night, in their tiny two-bedroom apartment, they housed Richard and Marjorie, me and Bill and Sewwandi's mother visiting from Sri Lanka. It was a fun evening, and the Sri Lankan food served that night was reminiscent of the country we had all left behind. They had their first child in May 2021.

Vasuki continued working as our Tamil teacher and my interpreter in Jaffna until she secured full time work at an all-girls school. Before long, health issues forced her and her husband, Mick, to return to the UK for treatment. I was unable to communicate with them for several years, but then found an email address for

Vasuki when I was seeking permission to include her in the memoir. We have re-established a warm connection.

My colleague, Sadhika and her husband, Mihir, are Facebook friends, just like Sandamali, my Sinhala teacher. We write notes to each other regularly.

Judgey, the tiny orange kitten we rescued in Sri Lanka passed away in July 2019. After a brief period of being unable to eat, followed by exploratory surgery, she succumbed to lymphoma. She was so loved because of her personality, but she was also a symbol, a touchstone to that other life in that far away land of serendipity.

And so, like Mr Winterfield in Wilkie Collins' story *The Black Robe*, it seems that I am at the end of my story, and it is time to make my disappearance.

Acknowledgements

It is with great pleasure that I can acknowledge some of the people and groups that have led to the publication of my first book. First, the inception of this story came after reading a newspaper article about Canadian University Services Overseas (CUSO), and the stories in this memoir are derived from the experience that CUSO International provided us. Without the support they provide to volunteers, it is doubtful we could have mustered the courage to venture out alone or return in one piece.

To my CUSO/VSO manager, Chandima Kulathunge, thank you for supporting my work and approving and funding all my projects. To USAID, who funded the work of my interpreter, Vasuki. Without that support, I could not have covered so much ground in my teaching.

No acknowledgement of this book would be complete without the support, love, camaraderie and friendship of the other CUSO/VSO volunteers in Sri Lanka between 2011 and 2012. It is not usual to have such a group of like-minded, fun loving, serious and dedicated volunteers from across the globe that, for the most part, genuinely enjoyed one another. For them, for their support and friendship, Bill and I are most grateful.

These volunteers are too numerous to mention here. However, Dr Kamal Kainth was instrumental in keeping us sane in the cold of Nuwara Eliya. I would be remiss to not acknowledge the Jaffna Family that included Dr Marcia Brophy, Jo Coombs, Mary Cuttle, and Ann Murray. We extended the Jaffna Family to include Gerd Buta and Mitsuko Nishimori, who were not with CUSO/VSO but became part of our family there. The friendship of these volunteers was critical during our year in Jaffna.

I wish to acknowledge Chamali Senanayake. She is pure goodness. She worked tirelessly with me to translate, to brainstorm, to plan, to teach me the culture, and to take care of me. I love her very much and will never forget her kindness to me and to others. She is a nurse and human being extraordinaire.

The stories contained in this memoir would still be scattered about my computer in blogs, bits of stories, notes, and pictures if not for the Cauldron. Although Donna Bishop and I had been colleagues at the hospital, I didn't know she was a writer until we both showed up at a local writers' conference. She sought permission for me to attend her writing group, The Cauldron.

My peers within this diverse group of writers are Donna Bishop, a novelist; Lissa Millar, a screenwriter; Nancy Van Veen, a travel writer; and Pete Smith, our resident poet. Their support and continuity in the group have been instrumental. I wish to acknowledge three members of my book club: Debi Adams, Margaret Abramzik and Leslie Hall who performed double duty as a focus group and proof readers. As well, I wish to thank two members of my hiking group, Cindy Huber and Brenda Boyd, businesswomen, who served and continue to serve as marketing consultants.

I wish to acknowledge my friend, Joan Gordon. Joan's husband, Jim, and my husband, Bill, were colleagues, and despite Joan and I knowing one another through this connection, we did not know we both aspired to write. More than twenty-five years ago, she showed up in the same writing class at the local university and we have been friends since. She continues to write and mentor my work.

I appreciated our visitors to Sri Lanka from Canada. To my daughters, Tanya and Lisa, who trekked over to share the experience with us and to reduce our homesickness. Your presence was a wonderful present, a touchstone to home. To my mother, Maybelle Nordick, who despite her age and her dislike of spicy foods, came to visit and enjoyed every minute. It was a pleasure to watch your delight.

To T.J., thank you for coming and giving us the pleasure of seeing you get sprayed by an elephant. To Jen Sheeley for visiting me twice. You have a way of making everything fun yet profound.

To Drs Ajith Navaratne, Daya Somasundaram, and S. Sivayokan. Your leadership, mentorship, and expertise assisted me in my role as a volunteer. You are helping not only your country but also the mentally ill and war affected of the world. I am most grateful for your support.

To our children, Richard, Tanya, Rob, Brett, Carla, Shelley, and Lisa. I know we left you at a busy time in your life. You were going to university, working, giving birth, and raising your own families without our support during those two years. Your independence during that time left us able to do something out of the ordinary.

I acknowledge and extend deep gratitude to my parents, Ed and Maybelle Nordick for their enduring love, support and encouragement that has enabled me to believe in myself.

Finally, to my husband, Bill. I want to acknowledge that whatever I want to do, you support me. I want a master's degree. Go for it. I want a PhD. Don't worry about the money. Go and get it. You want to volunteer with CUSO? So do I. Bill, you have been a wonderful life partner, always eager to embark on a journey. Thank you.

References

Enforced Disappearances in Sri Lanka. (24 November 2019). In *Wikipedia*.
https://en.wikipedia.org/wiki/Enforced_disappearances_in_Sri_Lanka

Collins, W. (1881) *The Black Robe*, UK: All The Year Round.

Dugard, M. (2001) *Farther than any man: The rise and fall of Captain James Cook*, New York: Washington Square Press.

Forster, E. M. (1924) *A Passage to India*, (Copyright: 1989). Montreal: Readers Digest Association, Inc.

Guastello, S. (1997). Science evolves: An introduction to nonlinear dynamics, psychology and life sciences. *Nonlinear dynamics, psychology and life sciences, 1*(1), 16. Retrieved from
http://www.societyforchaostheory.org/ndpls/editorial_1997.pdf

Hakgala Botanical Gardens. (29 November 2019) In *Wikipedia*
https://en.wikipedia.org/wiki/Hakgala_Botanical_Garden

Hoole, R., Somasundaram, D., Sritharan, K., Thiranagama, R. (1990) *The Broken Palmyra*, Claremont: CA. Available online at:
http://www.uthr.org/BP/Content.htm

Nallur Festival—A Magnificent Adoration of Lord Murugan. (25 July 2018) *TimeOut*. Retrieved from
https://www.timeout.com/sri-lanka/things-to-do/nallur-festival-a-magnificent-adoration-of-lord-murugan

Klodawsky, H. (2005) *No more tears sister: Anatomy of hope and betrayal* (Film). National Film Board of Canada. The first part is available at: https://www.youtube.com/watch?v=C803NOvmTqk

Ondaatje, M. (1982) *Running in the Family*, Toronto: McClelland and Stewart.

Rameez, R. (18 August 2018) The Real Line Room Experience: Through the eyes of an estate worker. *Roar Media*. Retrieved from http://roar.media/english/life/in-the-know/the-real-line-room-experience-through-the-eyes-of-an-estate-worker/

Sirilal, R. & Hull, C.B. (6 July 2010) Sri Lanka hardliners protest U.N. war crimes probe. *Reuters*. Retrieved from https://www.reuters.com/article/us-srilanka-un/sri-lanka-hardliners-protest-u-n-war-crimes-probe-idUSTRE6651MI20100706

Swamy, M.R.N. (2008) *Tigers of Lanka: From boys to guerrillas* (9th ed.), Colombo: Vijitha Yapa Publications.

Weiss, G. (2012) *The Cage: The fight for Sri Lanka and the last days of the Tamil Tigers*, London: Vintage Books.

Religion in Sri Lanka. (28 April 2020) In *Wikipedia*. https://en.wikipedia.org/wiki/Religion_in_Sri_Lanka

Indelible Reading Guide

1. **Voice**: A memoir is a first-person narrative. How would you describe the voice of the author? What characteristics of the author were made evident through her storytelling?
2. **Values**: By the author's own account, she was driven to volunteer with CUSO by strong values. What values do you think she held that made her want to volunteer? Did these values endure or change during the experience?
3. **Characterisation**: How does the character of Bill enhance the story? Chamali adds character to a real person in Sri Lanka. How did she assist the author?
4. **Style**: The author came from an academic background. Do you think that she was successful in bridging the gap between academic writing and narrative writing? Why or why not? What examples are evident where there is a clear break from academic writing?
5. **Location**: The author lived in two different locations in the story. How did the climate, the racial origin of the people and the environment impact her and her husband? Which location would you have preferred and why?
6. **Supervision**: The author struggled to bridge western therapeutic methods with culturally appropriate methods. Did she find a way to bridge the gap? What measures were taken? Was it sufficient? What do you think about western 'do-gooders' going to another country to provide a service?
7. **War**: The war impacted the people of Sri Lanka. In what way were the people impacted? Although, the war was over, did the war have an effect on the author? In what way?
8. **Murder**: There are two murders described in the book. How did those murders impact you? The author? The family members?

9. **Torture**: The author describes her research into the methods of torture and the treatment of torture victims. How did that impact you as the reader? PTSD is often a lasting effect of torture. How can therapy mitigate some of the effects of PTSD? What did you feel about her comparison of watching torture to pornography?

10. **Spirituality**: In the story, the author immediately makes is evident that spirituality is important to her. In what ways was her spirituality of assistance to her? Was it ever a hindrance? How did you feel about her relationship with Jesus?

11. **Emotion**: The author admits to tears many times. Was there a time in the story where the story provoked a powerful emotion in you? What emotion comes to mind and why?

Recommended Additional Resources List

Feedspot: https://blog.feedspot.com/volunteer_websites/

Canadian University Services Overseas: https://cusointernational.org

Developing World Connections: https://developingworldconnections.org

Global Work and Travel: https://globalworkandtravel.com/

Global Volunteers: https://globalvolunteers.org

Habitat for Humanity: https://habitat.ca/en/

National Film Board (2005). No More Tears Sister: anatomy of hope and betrayal: https://www.nfb.ca/film/no-more-tears-sister-anatomy-of-hope-and-betrayal/

Second Wind Volunteer: http://secondwindmovement.com/volunteer-websites/

Spark Ontario: https://www.sparkontario.ca

Peace Corps: https://www.peacecorps.gov

UN Volunteers: https://www.unv.org

Volunteer Abroad: https://www.goabroad.com/volunteer-abroad

Volunteer Forever: https://www.volunteerforever.com
VSO: https://www.vsointernational.org
Wikipedia: International Volunteering:
https://en.wikipedia.org/wiki/International_volunteering